First Steps in Medical Research

Volume 1

Medical Statistics & Scientific Publications Handling

2015

First edition

Cover & internal design: Mina Azer

First edition: 2015

First Printing: March 2015

ISBN-13: 978-1514351345

ISBN-10: 151435134X

FOCUS for capacity building solutions

In Cooperation with Society of Friends and Care of
Gastroenterology patients
1 Gawhar Al Sakaly St.
Mansoura, Al Dakahlya, Egypt.

www.focus4courses.blogspot.com

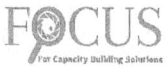 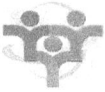

To my father and his sweet grand-daughter, as he led me through my first steps in my childhood and she dragged me back to its purity.

M. A.

To the gratitude towards my parents, the hope in my children, the support of my brother and sister, the help of my wife, and the love of them all.

H. H.

Authors' Biographies

Mina Azer got his MSc in surgery in 2013. He has a great passion for science yielded in his current research and publications. Between 2004 and 2014 he shared in more than 70 different training delivered to more than 2000 trainees about various topics such as: reproductive health, surgical skills, and medical research. He is currently working as a surgery specialist at the Egyptian Liver Research Institute and Hospital.

Hosam Hamed Has graduated from medical school in 2007. He got his MSc of surgery in 2012. He is currently an assistant lecturer of surgery in Gastroenterology Surgical Center - Mansoura University. Besides his aptitude for medical trainings he is interested in carrying out research projects that was published in various international journals.

Acknowledgment

This book could not be accomplished without the great and endless support of *Prof. Dr. Gamal Kamel El-Ebeidy,* professor of surgery – Mansoura University and a co-founder of the Society of Friends and Care of Gastroenterology patients – Mansoura.

The society hosted and funded 3 sessions of the Medical Students Research Grants. And based on the trainings delivered by the authors during these seasons this book was written.

The Authors

Contents

Preface

Do not read this book!

If you are not interested in understanding medical research process to be able to share in producing and consuming knowledge about the human body.

If you are already an expert in medical research. This book is for entry level medical researchers. It focuses on basics and lead you to a level in which you can: do simple research alone, do more complicated researches under supervision or be ready to complete your self-learning.

If you are – or want to be - a statistician. This book targets medical under/postgraduates. All topics and examples are tailored for them.

If you are seeking a family-size text book covering all topics of medical research. This book stops half way to the top, as we think that the rest can be found on other more sophisticated sources that won't be hard to understand anymore after you finish our book.

If you need to know the theory behind everything. This book is written by clinicians who do researches and train others to do so. We focused on how-to-do and what does this mean, but not on the mechanisms and boring equations. We are not that geeky, yet!

Part 1
Medical Statistics

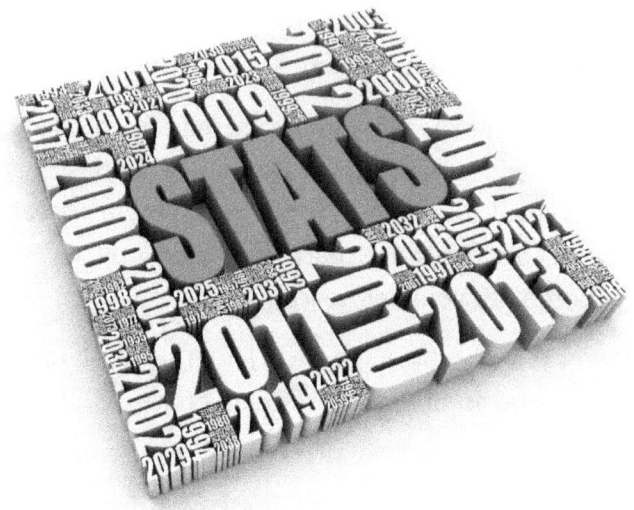

Train your mind. Starting with the basic concepts of probability, we will take you through the basic definitions of statistics to descriptive statistics. Then we will stress on the pillars of the statistical theory like the normal distribution and confidence interval. Now you will be ready to be introduced to the Null Hypothesis Significance Testing to start your adventure. We will give you one example for inferential methods which is linear correlation.

Chapter 1: Introduction

Medicine is being rewritten.

The knowledge about the human body, how it works and its diseases was accumulated throughout centuries, by the efforts of dedicated men and women, who depended on their sharp noticing and cognitive skills to observe the human body in health and sickness. They formed assumptions about the underlying mechanisms, then recommend reasonable maneuvers to adjust it during sickness. Starting from the middle of the 20th century a new model of thinking rose: Evidence Based Medicine.

Evidence based medicine was defined as: *"The use of mathematical estimates of the risk of benefit and harm, derived from high-quality research on population samples, to inform clinical decision-making in the diagnosis, investigation or management of individual patients[1]."*

Numbers never lie. Numbers are precise and emotionless. Numbers are trustable. That is why mathematical estimates through the statistical theory is now considered the most reliable way to generate our knowledge about the most scared entity in our universe: the human body. These estimates consider the balance of benefit and harm accompanying any medical intervention to justify its use. This is done by trying this intervention first on a population sample that is carefully selected to be able to

---

[1] Greenhalgh, Trisha (2010). How to Read a Paper: The Basics of Evidence-Based Medicine (4th Ed.). John Wiley & Sons. p. 1.

represent the entire population, then the sample is usually divided into 2 groups: cases (the people who will receive the medical intervention under investigation), and controls (people who are exactly similar to the case group except they won't receive the medical intervention). This serves the purpose of ensuring that the effect that would appear within the cases group is only due to the intervention by isolating any possible confounder. After that, results are compared using statistical tests to measure the benefit or harm appeared after the intervention. Then recommendations can be driven from these results to help the clinical decision makers, which is the ultimate goal of clinical research.

Although modern medicine is -to some extend- a *Western science*. It is well known that it has its roots in the medieval medicine, which is in turn can be considered as *Arabian science*. Even the idea of Evidence based practice has shadows in the ancient manuscripts of Arab scientists. Testing medical interventions for efficacy has existed since the time of Avicenna's The Canon of Medicine in the 11th century[2].

Studying medical statistics is the only way to share in *generating* science instead of just *consume* it. Although it is a demanding quest, its benefits cannot be underestimated. It enables doctors and health care givers to better understand the origins of medical interventions they use with their patients. Also they can judge different data regarding incidence of diseases, risks of maneuvers and prognostic

[2] Brater DC, Daly WJ (May 2000). "Clinical pharmacology in the Middle Ages: principles that presage the 21st century". *Clin. Pharmacol. Ther.* 67 (5): 447–50

assumptions in a more enlightened vision. With more advanced levels of knowledge, they will be able to perform their own research about the crucial issues facing them during their clinical practice.

The best way of dealing with studying medical statistics is to consider it as a new language you are about to learn. Languages are better to be learnt by immersion, like the first language you learned as a child, remember that it just took you 18 to 24 month to understand and speak a language without having lessons or taking exams. This is because you were immersed in the language, surrounded by expressions and words in all times, and trying to use it in every situation. First you made a lot of mistakes, but as days went on, you improved your skills till you are now able to use the language without even thinking. The same concept could be applied to medical statistics. You must know that it will take you time, trials and mistakes till you are able to use it. The key factor that you should keep trying to use it.

(980 – 1037 AD)

Writer

Avicenna was a Persian polymath who is regarded as one of the most significant thinkers and writers of the Islamic Golden Age. Of the 450 works he is known to have written, around 240 have survived, including 150 on philosophy and 40 on medicine[3].

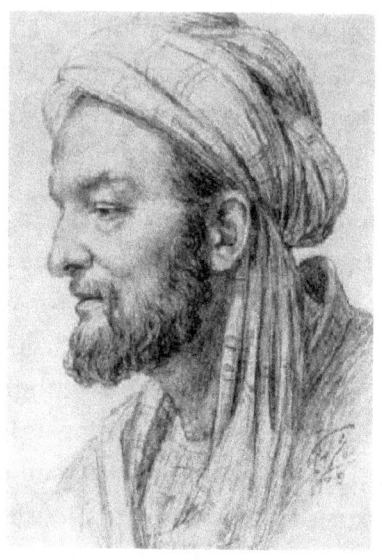

---

[3] Wikipedia

Chapter 2: Basics of Probability

Learning objectives:
- What is probability?
- Methods of calculation of probability
- Rules of addition and multiplication

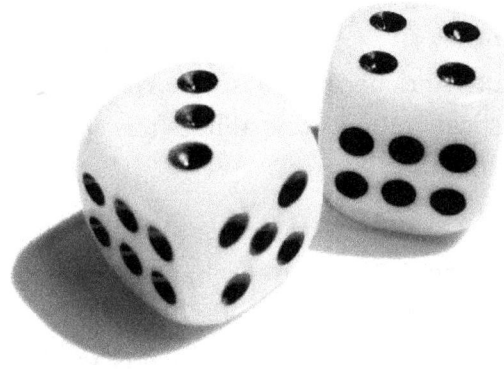

Probability is a measure of uncertainty. It is a measure of the chance of a given event to occur. This event can be an *everyday life event*, like the probability of meeting a friend by chance while walking home or the probability of getting a tail or head while flipping a coin. It can be also a *clinical event,* like the probability of recurrence of a certain tumor after surgical excision. This event is not certain as the tumor could recur or not, even if there is a high chance that it would recur (as high as 99%). Still there is a 1% chance that it would not recur. And here comes the role of clinical research and statistical methods to estimate this chance and represent it with a number.

On the other hand, inevitable events or impossible events are both outside the scope of probability, and in turn outside the scope of clinical research. For example the chance that human being would die is 100%, it is a certainty, so you cannot justify a research that try to ask the question of: *what is the percent of cancer patients who would eventually die?* As they all will, and the answer of your question is already known. But you can lead a research on *the percent of cancer patient who would die after 1 year of the surgical resection.* This is a valid research as there is a chance that those patient would die within 1 year or live longer, and that is what is known as the 1 year survival. Similarly, impossible events are outside the scope of research.

Probability is expressed as a positive number that lies between zero and one. If it is equal to zero, then the event cannot occur. If it is equal to one, then the event must occur. This number is calculated as a fraction in which the nominator is the event that you would like to calculate its probability, and the denominator is the number of all possible events that could happen.

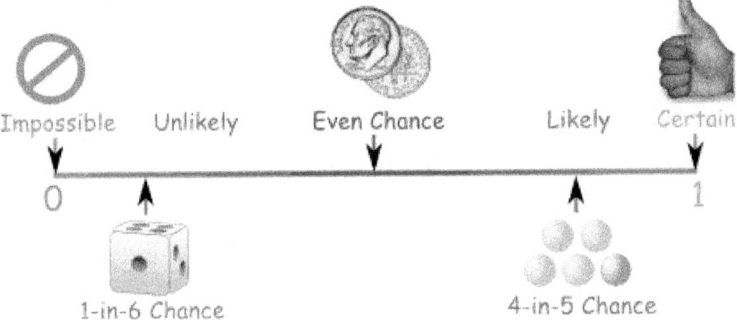

For example, what is the probability of getting a head while flipping a coin?

You can say by common sense that there is a chance of 50% that I would get a head, but how this figure was calculated?

The fraction is formed as following:

Nominator: the calculated event = 1 (it means it is 1 event that we want to calculate which is "heads" would appear)

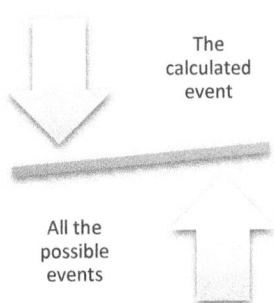

<u>Denominator:</u> All the possible events = 2 (it means there are only 2 events could happen, either a "head" would appear or a "tail" – there is no other possibilities)

So, the fraction is ½ = 0.5 = 50%.

And that is how probability estimates are expressed. Any positive number between 0 and 1 is a fraction calculated the same way. And a certainty is expressed as 1 or 100% from the fraction 1/1 that means there is only one possible event would happen which is the one we are calculating its probability. And in the same way, the impossible event is expressed as 0 or 0% from the fraction 0/1.

Calculation of probability

There are 3 ways to calculate the fraction of probability for any given event.

1- **Subjective method**— which represents our personal degree of belief that the event will occur. It a rough estimation and varies from person to person. It is used only in our daily life but not in clinical research.

Depends on personal judgment and available information about the event under consideration.

2- **Priori method**—which requires knowledge of the theoretical model, called the probability distribution. For example the coin toss is a model where there is only 2 possible events with the same chance to happen (provided that the coin is fair, i.e. without any variation in its shape that favors its fall on either sides.

Depends on a known model.

3- **Frequentist method**— which is the proportion of times the event would occur if we were to repeat the experiment a large number of times. It is the most widely used method in clinical research when no certain rule or pattern is known.

For example, clinical research estimated that the most common etiology of hepatocellular carcinoma (HCC) is viral hepatitis (HCV or HBV) where 90% of patients with HCC have also viral hepatitis. This can be also stated as: "the probability of a patient with HCC to have also viral hepatitis is 0.9". How was that calculated?

There is no place for guessing in clinical research, so subjective method is omitted. And there is no known model to build on it using the priori method, as we do not know if the chances of the patient to have viral hepatitis or no are equal (i.e. it is not a fair coin). So the solution is the Frequentist method.

Let's assume that every HCC patient is a coin flip or toss. If he has viral hepatitis, the flip is heads. If he has not viral hepatitis, the flip is tails. Let's then flip the coin 100 times to try to observe a pattern. This means that we will examine 100 different HCC patients. We will find that the heads (viral hepatitis) appeared in 90 patients (coin flips) and the tails (no viral hepatitis) appeared in 10 patients. So the fraction of the event we want to calculate for = 90 over the total number of events = 100. So the probability is 90/100 = 0.9 = 90%.

Depends on the accuracy of observation and the number of trial (sample size).

Rules of probability

When trying to calculate the probability of 2 events to happen together there are 2 rules: Addition rule and Multiplication rule. You can either add the probabilities of each of them or multiply them. This depends on the type of these events for being either mutually exclusive or independent events.

Mutually exclusive events: each event precludes the other, i.e. both events cannot happen in the same time. E.g. Heads and tails of a coin or 1, 2, 3,4,5,6 on a dice roll. You can either get a head or a tail but never both, or you can get 1 or 4 when you roll a dice but never both.

- The sum of their probabilities is always one.

- Addition rule: is used to calculate the probabilities of 2 or more events of this type – if the probability of getting 1 in a dice is 1/6 and getting 4 is 1/6 too, so the probability of getting 1 or 4 is 1/6 + 1/6 = 2/6

Independent events: the occurrence of one event is not contingent on the other. They can both occur at the same time. E.g. Gender (m/f) and heads/tails of a coin. Let's suppose that a group of people are tossing coins, they are 5 males and 5 females, and you are going to select one of them randomly (while closing your eyes). The probability of choosing a female and that she gets a tail in her coin toss are 2 independent events, as they can both happen in the same time. But the probability of choosing a female and a male is a mutually exclusive event.

- The sum of their probabilities is not one.

- <u>Multiplication rule:</u> is used to calculate the probabilities of 2 or more events of this type. The probability of choosing a female and that she gets a tail in her coin toss is calculated by multiplying the probability of choosing a female time the probability of getting a tail.

  - Choosing a female is determined by *Frequentist method*, 5 female/10 people = 5/10 = ½.
  - Getting a tail is determined by priori method as a model of the coin is known, it is equal ½
  - The probability of both events together is ½ X ½ = ¼

Note that expressing 2 mutually exclusive events is done by saying OR, while independent events can be expressed by saying AND.

Summary

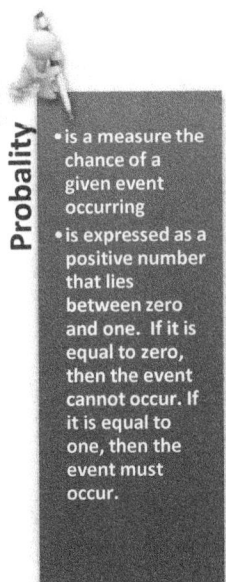

Probality

- is a measure the chance of a given event occurring
- is expressed as a positive number that lies between zero and one. If it is equal to zero, then the event cannot occur. If it is equal to one, then the event must occur.

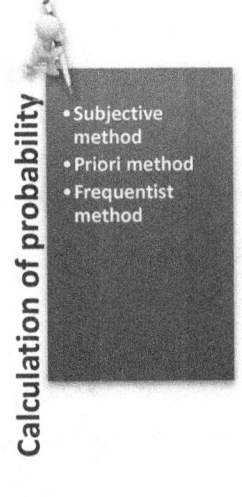

Calculation of probability

- Subjective method
- Priori method
- Frequentist method

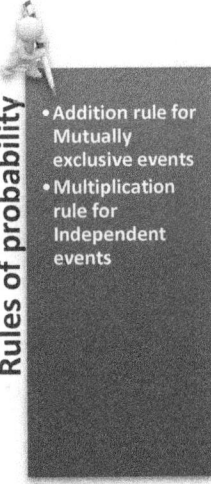

Rules of probability

- Addition rule for Mutually exclusive events
- Multiplication rule for Independent events

Chapter 3: Basic Statistical Definitions

Learning objectives:

- Data
- Variables; definition and types
- Samples and population
- Major branches of statistics

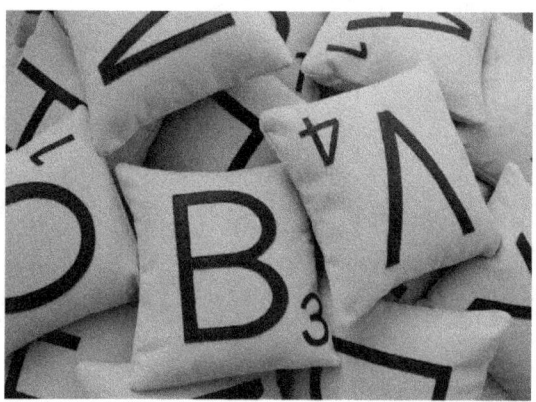

Data

Is the lowest level of abstraction from which information and then knowledge are derived. *For example*, the arterial blood pressure of a certain person is 120/80. This is a *datum* (singular of data). The average of arterial blood pressure of 1000 normal person was 120/80. This is an *information*. Assuming that the normal arterial blood pressure is 120/80 in human beings, and knowing when it is high (hypertension) or low (hypotension) is *knowledge*.

Variables vs. Constants

Variables can take on multiple values. In contrast, a constant has only one value. An example for variable is the arterial blood pressure as it can take different values among different persons or even in the same person from time to time. But normal arterial blood pressure is a constant as it is always be 120/80 for any time or situation.

- Arterial blood pressure = 120/80 or 155/95 or 100/65 etc., so it is a variable.
- Normal arterial blood pressure = 120/80 only, so it is a constant.

Medical statistics and clinical research deals mainly with variables as they show variations that could be measured, compared or altered in different situations. While constant values once determined, they are out of the scope of clinical research.

Types of variables

1. Cracking classification

- <u>Discrete variable</u> e.g. gender male or female (no values in between those two values)
- <u>Continuous variable</u> e.g. age 1, 2 year (there are potential values in between like 1.5, 1.75 etc.)

2. Levels of measurement precision classification - Scale

1. <u>Nominal scale</u>

Allows for only qualitative classification. That is because they can be measured only in terms of whether the individual items belong to some distinctively different categories or not, but we cannot quantify or even rank order those categories.

Typical examples of nominal variables are gender, race, color, city of birth, etc.

2. <u>Ordinal scale</u>

Allows us to rank order the items we measure in terms of which has less and which has more of the quality represented by the variable, but still it does not allow us to say "how much more."

A typical example of an ordinal variable is the socioeconomic status of families.

3. <u>Interval scale</u>

Allows us not only to rank the items, but also to quantify and compare the sizes of differences between them. For example, temperature, as measured in degrees Fahrenheit or Celsius, constitutes an interval scale

Zero is a value and does not mean absence of the quality. For example, zero degree Celsius does not mean absence of temperature as there is lower degree of temperature like -1, -3 etc.

4. Ratio scale

Are very similar to interval variables; in addition to all the properties of interval variables, they feature an identifiable absolute zero point, thus they allow for statements such as x is two times more than y.

Typical examples of ratio scales are measures of time or space

Zero means absence of the quality – zero distance means no distance.

*Most statistical data analysis procedures do not distinguish between the interval and ratio properties of the measurement scales. Software for statistical analysis like SPSS assign both ratio and interval variable as: **Scale variables***

3. Qualitative classification

- Independent (predictor variables): The variables that enters the study to measure their effect on other variables.
- Dependent (outcome variables): The variables that are investigated during the study to determine the effect elected upon them by the independent variables.

Unlike the previous 2 classifications of variables, this classification does not depend on the nature of the variable itself, but on its rule in the study.

For example, if we want to determine the effect of the duration of surgery on the incidence of wound infection, duration of surgery will be the independent variable, as during analysis we do not build a relation between it and any other variables. The dependent variable will be the incidence of wound infection as it depends on a previous variable which is the duration of surgery. In another scenario, if we are investigating the effect of wound infection on the hospital stay, the incidence of wound infection will be the independent variable, while the duration of hospital stay will be the dependent variable. But in both scenarios, the duration of surgery and the hospital stay will remain a continuous, ratio variable (time measured in minutes, hours or days) and the incidence of wound infection will remain a discrete, nominal variable (yes/no – weather there is wound infection or not).

The effect of the duration of surgery on the incidence of wound infection → **duration of surgery** — independent — continuous, ratio → **incidence of wound infection** — dependent — discrete, nominal

The effect of wound infection on the hospital stay → **incidence of wound infection** — independent — discrete, nominal → **hospital stay** — dependent — continuous, ratio

Sample vs. population

Sample: a subset of the population on which we perform our study.

Population: the entire collection of cases to which we want to generalize on by performing our study on a sample selected from it.

Statistic: a numerical measure that describes a characteristic of a sample.

Parameter: a numerical measure that describes a characteristic of a population.

Example:

We want to determine the average height of Egyptian males at the age of 18 years.

We will have 2 options, either to gather all the Egyptian males at the age of 18, then measure their heights and determine their average, or if we don't have the time or the resources to do so, we can just take a random sample of them, say 1000 guys, measure their heights and determine the average. The number we get is the average of the 1000 guys (our *sample*) but we can assume that it represent the average height of all Egyptian males at the age of 18 (our *population*). The average height of the sample is the *statistic* that we assume to represent the average of the population, which is the *parameter*.

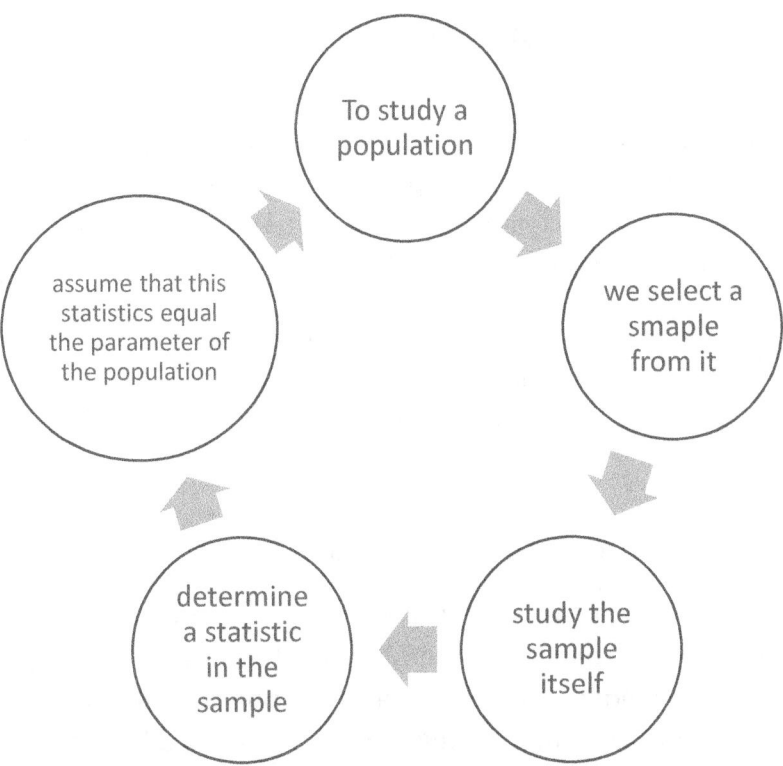

Types of statistics

o **Descriptive statistics:**

Procedures that organize and summarize the data. The aim of descriptive statistics is to describe any given set of data in the shortest form possible. It does not deal with populations and samples. It just describe the sample itself. It depends on 3 basic components:

- Measure of central tendency
- Measure of variance
- Graphical illustration

o **Inferential statistics:**

Procedures that allow for generalizations about population parameters based on sample statistics. Through these methods we can draw conclusions about the population we study through information gained from the sample. Its 2 main branches are:

- Correlational: Examine relationships among existing variables.
- Experimental: studying the effect of new variables added during an experiment or a clinical trial.

For example: knowing the average height of 1000 Egyptian males at the age of 18 is a descriptive statistics, but being able to say that this average height we got from the sample is equal to the average height of all Egyptian males at the age of 18 (population) is an inferential statistics.

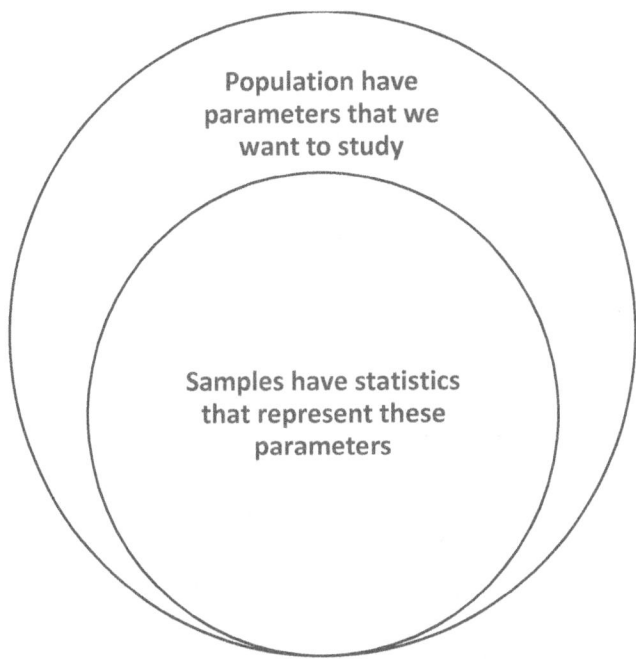

Summary

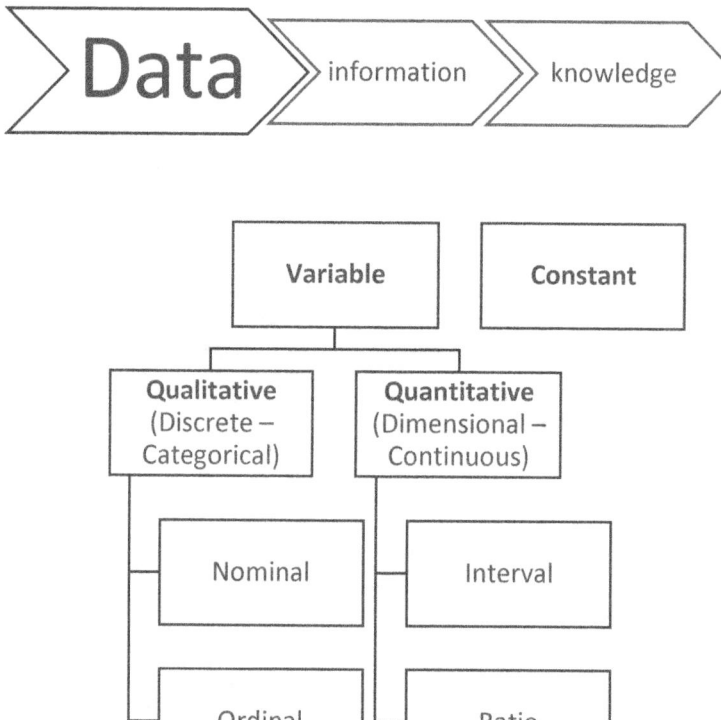

The amount of knowledge we get from each type of variables

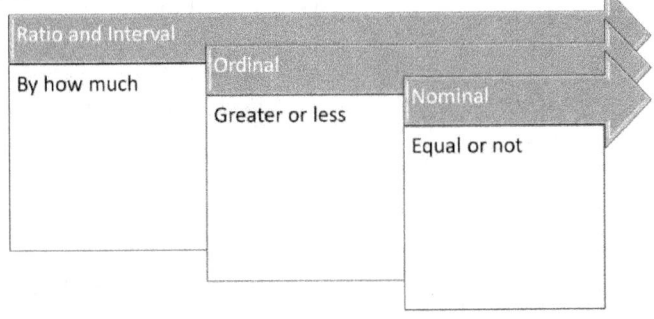

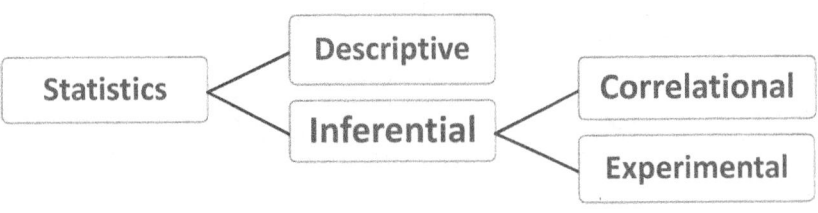

Chapter 4: Descriptive Statistics

Learning objectives:

- Measurement of central tendency: mode, median & mean
- Measurement of variance: range, percentile, variance & standard deviation
- Graphical illustration: histogram & whisker-box plot
- The concept of outliers

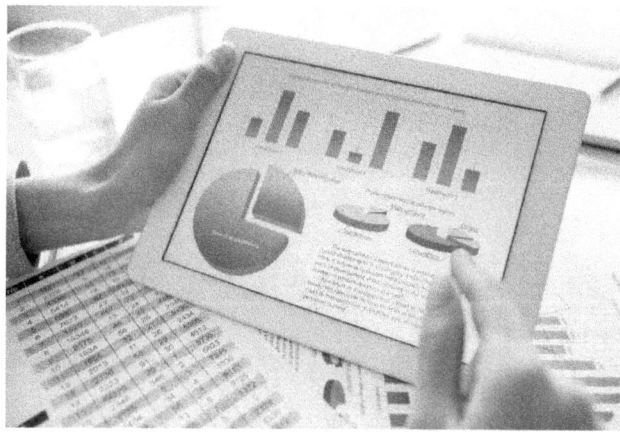

As mentioned before, the ultimate goal of descriptive statistics is to summarize the information we can get from a set of data into the shortest form possible. As in language, summarizing is an important skill that does not just enables you to cut long text short, but it shows how deep do you understand that text.

When summarizing a text you should keep a delicate balance between decreasing the number of words and keeping the meaning untouched. Of course you might lose some minor ideas, figures of speech or hidden meanings, but on the other hand you get a text that is easily understood, can be quickly processed and does not consume your hard drive storage space.

In this chapter we will go through the process of summarizing statistical data through the techniques of descriptive statistics. We will discuss its 2 main components in details; central tendency and variance. The third component; the graphical illustration will be dealt with throughout this and the next chapters according to the appropriate use of every graph.

The idea of descriptive statistics

Suppose that you have a set of data representing the ages of 20 persons. You don't have any additional ideas about those persons, and you were asked to draw as many conclusions as possible from these data.

The first step, you should take a good look on the data. At the first glance, you can conclude they are mostly young people. This looks like an easy task because there only 20 persons, but what if your data sheet goes on till thousands of entries. You will need the following tools.

Name	Age	Name	Age
A	15	K	23
B	17	L	24
C	23	M	23
D	28	N	19
E	19	O	22
F	49	P	26
G	26	Q	23
H	18	R	29
I	27	S	15
J	52	T	18

If you were asked to choose one number to represent the whole set of 20 numbers, what number would you choose? The largest, the smallest or the middle number? I think by common sense you will choose the middle number. And this is the first tool you should use, which is the central tendency.

Central tendency means: where the center of your data set lies. Is it around 23 years, more or less? It is like saying that the number 23 is the best number to describe the whole set of numbers as it lies in the center of all data points.

But even if we agreed that the number 23 can represent each person best, we will find that it would not fit for all data points. Although for persons: C, K, L and O the age is very close or equal to 23, persons like A are too young or like F and J are too old to be represented by 23. We will need another value to describe this data set.

This value is the measure of variance, which tells us by how much each point of data (age of a person) is higher or lower than the center of the data that we agreed upon above.

In conclusion, for each set of data consists of as many as hundreds or thousands of numbers, we can describe those data by 2 numbers only: one for the center of the data (central tendency) and the other for the variation across the set of data (variance).

Like in a map, describing a data set needs 2 coordinates: central tendency and variance. Stating one without the other is like describing a location with altitude only, will lead to nowhere.

Measurement of Central tendency

Mode - Median - Mean

Mode

It is the value that occurs most frequently in a distribution of the set of data.

How to calculate: count the number of occurrence of every value, the highest frequency is the mode. In the previous example of the ages of 20 persons the mode was 23 as 4 persons had this age.

Mode may be:

- Unimodal: when the data have one mode, i.e. there is one value that occurred most frequently.
- Bimodal: when the data have two modes, i.e. when there are 2 values occurred nearly at the same frequency in the set of data. E.g. the bimodal distribution of the age of onset of symptoms of ulcerative colitis (UC). Studies found that UC can start at any age, but most frequently the age of patients was observed to be either in the second or fifth decade of life.
- Multimodal: when the data have more than two modes.

Mode is more useful in dealing with nominal variables, where it is the only way to determine their central tendency.

Median

It is the value that lies exactly midway in the frequency distribution of the set of data.

How to calculate: arrange the values in ascending or descending order, keep repeated values in place.

If the number of data points is an *odd number*: take the middle one to be the median. If the number of data points is an even number: take sum of the 2 middle values and divide it over 2 (the average of the 2 middle values), the result is the median.

The importance of the median that it lies in the middle, in other words in the 50th percentile of the data, this means that exactly half of the data points have values less than the median, and half have values greater.

Mean (arithmetic average)

It is the sum of all observations (data points) divided by the number of observations. It is the most important and informative measure of central tendency.

How to calculate:
$$\frac{\Sigma x}{n}$$

Sum of all data points

Number of data points

Example:

Calculate the mode, median and mean for the following set of data:

2	15	5	8	12	6	5	12	12	10

Mode = 12 (occurred 3 times)

Then arrange the data points in descending or ascending order

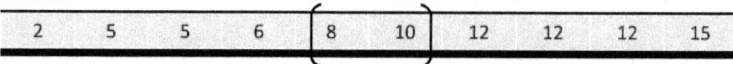

| 2 | 5 | 5 | 6 | 8 | 10 | 12 | 12 | 12 | 15 |

Since this set of data consists of 10 points (even number), then to get the median you should divide the sum of the 2 middle values (5th & 6th) by 2

Median = (8 + 10)/2 = 18/2 = 9

Mean = the sum divided by the number of data points = $\sum x/n$ = 87/10 = 8.7

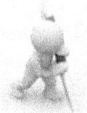

Notice that the mean and median in this set are close to each other (9 & 8.7). While the mode is much higher (12). when dealing with continuous (scale) variables, mean and median are more representative.

Histogram – Graphical illustration

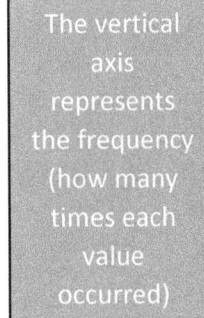

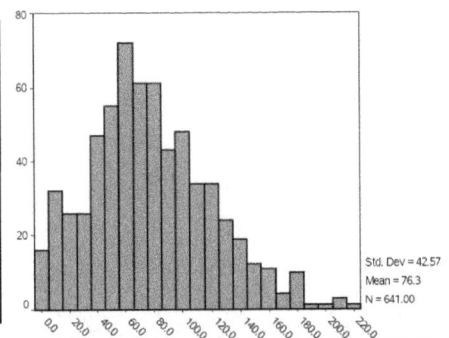

The horizontal axis represents the values

The histogram is an illustration of the frequency of occurrence of each value in the data set as in the above figure.

Histogram shapes:

- Bell-shaped, which represents the normal distribution (discussed later), simply it means that most values are in the middle, or near the mean and few values are on both extremes, either very high or very low *(e.g. IQ or Hemoglobin concentration)*, we can assume that IQ is bell-shaped on histograms, as if we illustrated the IQ of 1000 persons we mostly will find that most people have average IQ (between 110 and 130), few have very high IQ (genius) and few have very low IQ (mentally retarded).

- Skewed (positive) right: it means that few variable are found on the right (positive side) *(e.g. annual income)* we can assume that all people have annual income of at least 10 LE/month – and half people have at least 1000 LE/month – few people have 10,000 LE /month and very few have income of 100,000 LE/month.

- Skewed (negative) left: on the other hand when the few values are found on the left (negative) side *(e.g. score on an easy exam)* most students will get high marks (positive or right side values) but few students will insist on failure and get low marks (negative or left side values) despite the easy exam.

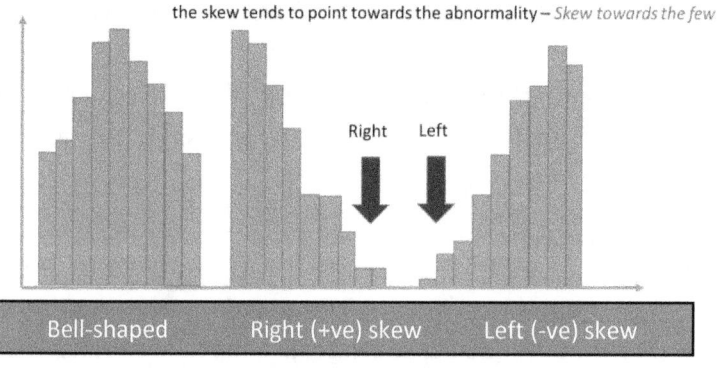

the skew tends to point towards the abnormality – *Skew towards the few*

Right   Left

| Bell-shaped | Right (+ve) skew | Left (-ve) skew |

Outliers

An outlier is an observation which does not appear to belong with the other data points. It may be too high or too low on the scale of measurement of the variable.

Outliers can arise because of a measurement or recording errors or because of equipment failure during an experiment, etc. Also an outlier might be indicative of a sub-population, e.g. an abnormally low or high value in a medical test could indicate presence of an illness in those patients.

Outliers should be:

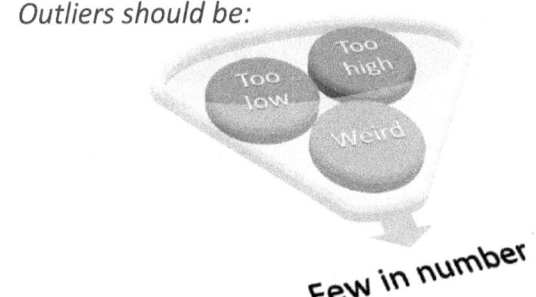

Few in number

Both skew and outliers can distort the values of mean of any given variable rendering it an unreliable representation of the central tendency of that variable.

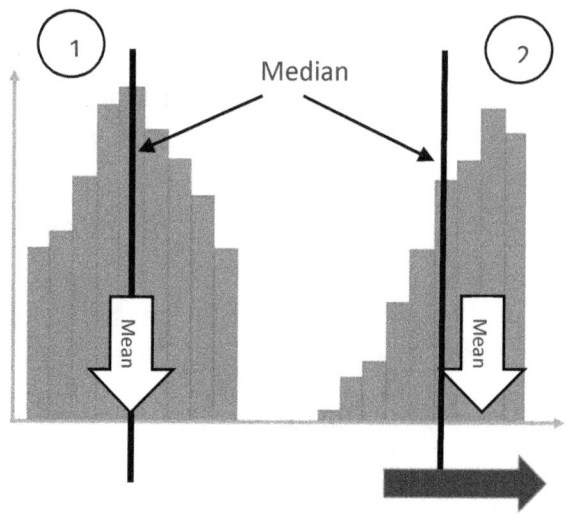

As we can see in the above figure, in a bell shaped histogram (1): both mean and median are found in the center of the histogram, this means that the number that the mean represents is nearly equal to the median, so the mean here is a good representation of the center of this variable. But in Right skewed histogram (2): the median remains in the center but the mean is dragged towards the higher values in the left side of the histogram (opposite to the direction of the skew).

The same effect can be noticed with outliers, an outliers with an unusually high (positive) value will drag the mean towards the positive direction but it well leave the median untouched.

Type	Advantages	Disadvantages	Uses
Mean	• Uses all data • Mathematically manageable	• Distorted by outliers and skew	• interval scales • normal distribution
Median	• Not distorted by outliers and skew	• Does not use all data • Not mathematically manageable	• interval or ordinal scales
Mode	• Defining modal distribution	• Does not use all data • Not mathematically manageable • Could be absent (if every value occurred only once)	• Nominal

45

Measurements of Variance

Range – Percentile - Variance - Standard deviation

Range

It is the difference between the largest and the smallest observations in the data set. It defines where the data set begins and ends.

While it is not the most informative measurement of variation across the data set, it gives us a glimpse on how variable are the data. *For example*, if a given data set had a median of 10 and range of 4, so we can assume that the largest number is 12 and the lowest is 8. So all the data are aggregated around the median, and the median is really representative of the data. But if in the same data, the range was 20, the highest value will be 20 and the lowest will be zero. So, the median here (10) is not very representative of the data.

Narrow range leads to the assumption that the median is a good representative of the data set, and vice versa.

Percentile

The *Median* divides a distribution into two halves. 50% of the values are above and 50% are below the median.

The *first and third quartiles* (denoted as Q1 and Q3) are defined as follows:

- 25% of the data lie below Q1 (and 75% is above Q1),
- 25% of the data lie above Q3 (and 75% is below Q3)

The *inter-quartile range (IQR)* is the difference between the first and third quartiles, i.e. IQR = Q3- Q1

The percentile can be considered as the further details of the range, While the range itself tells us where our data set begins and ends, the percentile shows us how the data are distributed within this range.

For example; a range of age of 30 persons can be 15 to 40. We cannot give any assumption based on this alone, but if the range tills us that the Q3 is 16, then we can assume that 75% of those persons are between 15 and 16 years, we can guess that this group are a classroom in high school with their teacher counted with them aged 40 years (by the way, the teacher's age here is an outlier).

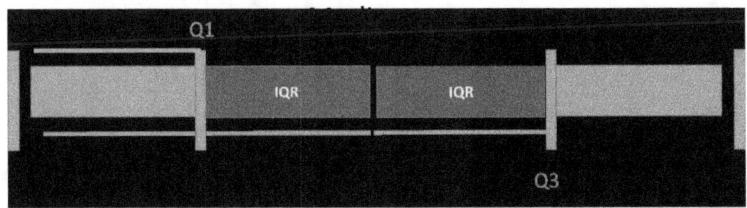

Box-whisker plots – Graphical illustration

They portray a five-numbers summary of the data:

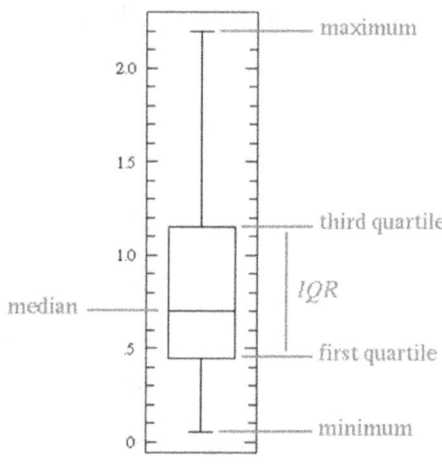

- Minimum
- Q1
- Median
- Q3
- Maximum

They represent the data as a box (for the IQR) and a line (for the Q1 & Q4) then suspected outliers are identified separately as a dot.

It helps in spotting the outliers by: Re-defining the upper and lower limits (fences) of the boxplots (the whisker lines) as:

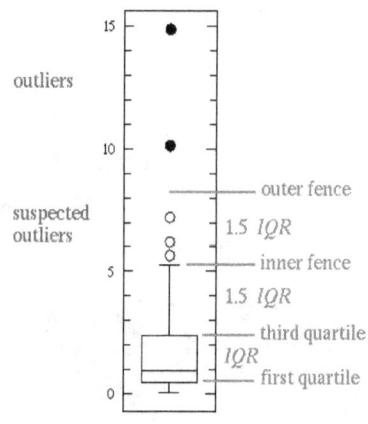

✓ Lower limit = Q1-1.5 X IQR
✓ Upper limit = Q3+1.5 X IQR

If a data point is less than the lower limit or more than the upper limit, the data point is considered to be an outlier.

Variance and Standard Deviation (SD)

48

Deviation of a value is the distance between this value and the mean, or in other words: the amount of its deviation from the center.

Variance: average squared deviation of all possible observations from a sample mean. Or it is the arithmetic mean of the squared deviations from the sample mean.

The logical meaning of variance that it is the amount of variation within the sample. The first step to calculate this variation is to set a middle (reference) point on the scale of the data to relate the variation to it. This point is the *Mean*. Variance tells us if our data is variable from the mean or nearly equal to it, and if variable, by how much?

2	15	5	9	12	8	5	12	12	10

In the above example, the mean = 9

The variation of each datum from the mean is calculated from subtracting the mean from this value. This variation is called the deviation. So, for the value 12 the deviation is $12 - 9 = 3$, for the value 9 (the 4th one) the deviation $= 9 - 9 = 0$, or it is not deviated from the mean, etc. if we want to calculate the variation across all data point we should calculate the average (mean) of all deviations.

But if we tried to get the sum of all deviations and divide them by the number of values, we will always get a result = Zero. That is because the numbers above mean will have positive deviations, equals to mean with zero deviations and below the mean gives negative deviations. So in order to get a positive number we will calculate the square of the deviation instead.

So variance (S^2) could be expressed by this equation:

$$s^2 = \frac{\sum\limits_{i=1}^{n}(x_i - \bar{x})^2}{n-1}$$

Note that variance is a square too, so the result of this equation is much higher than the real average deviation.

In order to get the real average deviation we calculate **standard deviation (s)** which is: positive square root of the variance. It can be considered as a "typical" distance from the mean.

Properties of the standard deviation (s):

- $s \geq 0$, and only equals 0 if all observations are equal.
- s increases with the amount of variation around the mean.
- s depends on the units of the data (e.g. measure euro vs. $).
- Like mean, it is affected by outliers.

Small standard deviation: observations are clustered tightly around the mean.

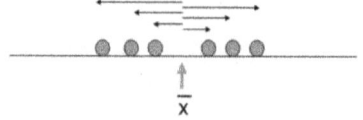

Large standard deviation: observations are scattered widely around the mean.

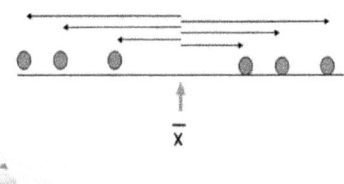

$$\overline{x}$$

To express any variable properly you must state its mean and SD in form of:

Mean ± SD

For example: the platelet count of the CBC of 100 patient was: 250 ± 90

	Advantage	Disadvantage
Range	easy	Does not use all data (only 2) Affected by outliers
percentile	Identify outliers Unaffected by skew	Does not use all data. Not algebraically defined
Variance	Use all data Algebraically defined	Affected by outliers – skew Units are squared (m^2 for distance)
Standard deviation	Use all data Algebraically defined Same unit of the data Easily interpreted	Affected by outliers - skew

Summary

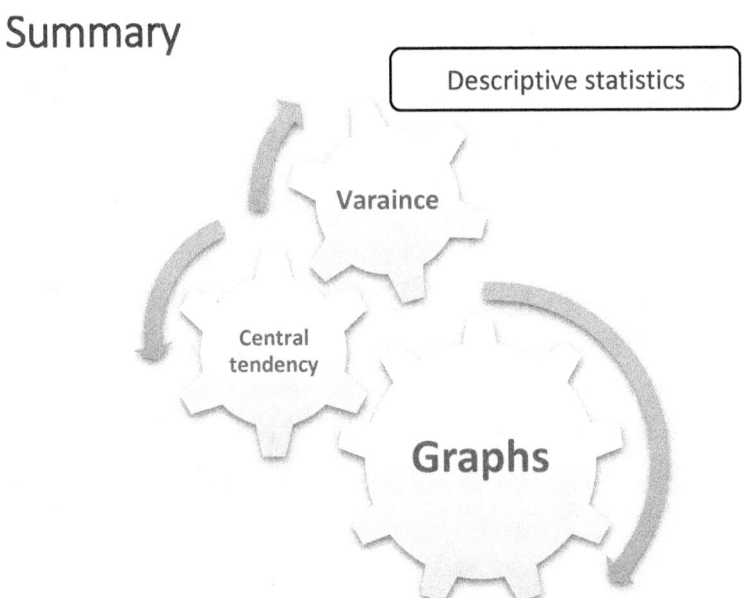

Descriptive statistics

Varaince

Central tendency

Graphs

Central tendency

Mode

- It is the value that occurs most frequently in a distribution of the set of data.

Mean

- It is the sum of all observations (data points) divided by the number of observations.

Median

- It is the value that lies exactly midway in the frequency distribution of the set of data.

Variation

Range

- It is the difference between the largest and the smallest observations in the data set.

Percentile

- Points on the scale before which a certain percentage of data exist.

Variance

- Average squared deviation of all possible observations from a sample mean.

Standard deviation

- Positive square root of the variance. It can be considered as a "typical" distance from the mean.

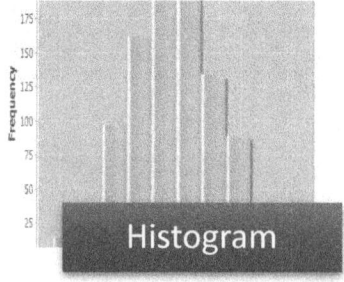

Histogram

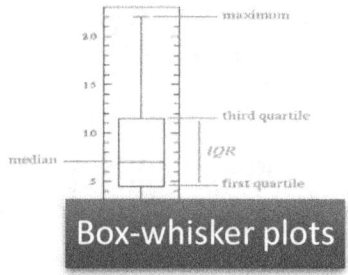

Box-whisker plots

Chapter 5: Normal Distribution

Learning objectives:

- Definition and properties of normal distribution
- Probability calculation of normal distribution
- Skewness and kurtosis

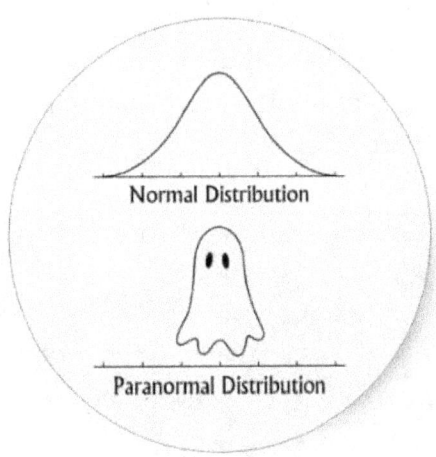

The word "Normal" in language carries the meaning of "common" also. It is obvious that any variation in nature looks like a spectrum with different grades within, this spectrum usually have a common type and rare or extreme types. For example, the height of people. If you measured the height of a lot of people, you will notice that the majority of them are between 160 and 180 cm, but few are taller and few are shorter, and the number of people of a height of 190 are less than of the height 180, and in turn fewer are of a height of 200, and very few are 210 etc. and the same applies to the shorter people, few are short, fewer are shorter and the fewest are suffering from dwarfism.

This is the main idea behind the normal distribution, that the middle of the scales are the more common and the extremes in both sides are rare.

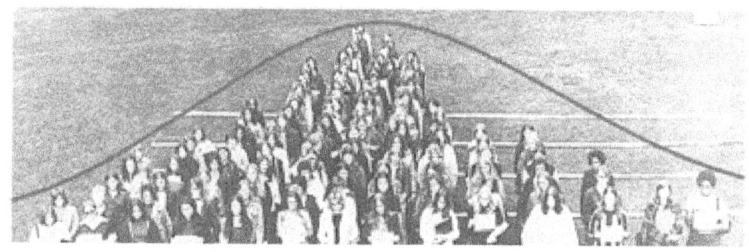

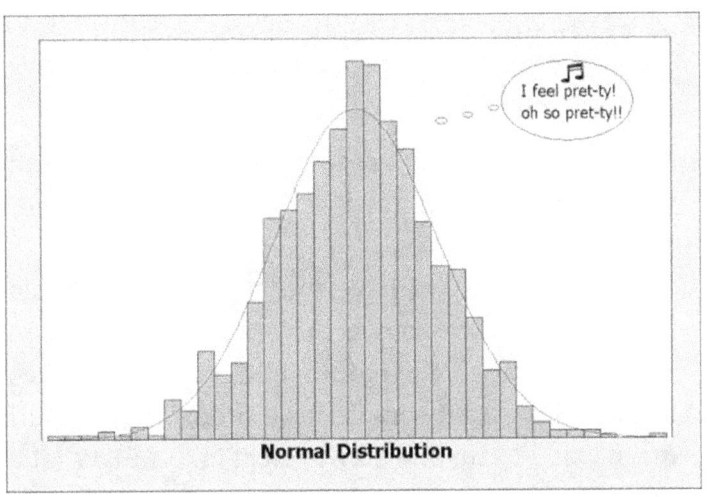

Normal Distribution

The normal distribution when plotted on a histogram will have *the following properties:*

- *Bell shaped curve* with highest point at mean.
- *Symmetric* about mean.
- *Unimodal.*
- *Continuous* distribution, there is a probability to find a value between any 2 given values. You can find a guy with a height of 172.444 cm between 2 guys of 172.443 and 172.445 cm and so on.
- Approaches horizontal axis *but never touches it*, as there will be always a theoretical tiny probability that you can find a guy of a height of 3 m or 100 m etc. touching the horizontal line (the Zero on the vertical axis) means that the probability is zero.

Probabilities according to Standard Deviation (SD)

Another important property of the variable with normal distribution that it is possible to link the percentage of cases to the SD.

For example, we have the heights of a sample of 100 persons, and we know that the height is a normally distributed variable in nature, also we confirmed (as we will see later) that our sample have a normal distribution. The mean was 170 cm and SD was 5 cm (170 ± 5). What does this mean?

It means that the center of our sample (the most common height) is 170 cm. and the average of the difference between all data (persons) and the 170 cm is 5 cm. So we can find persons measured 175, 177, 160 and 165 etc.

The rule of probabilities of a normally distributed variables states that:
- ✓ Within the first 2 SD (between +5 & -5) there are 68% of the cases
- ✓ Within the second 2 SD (between +10 & -10) there are 95% of the cases
- ✓ Within the third 2 SD (between +15 & -10) there are 99.3% of the cases

In other words, in the variable of mean 170 and SD 5, 68% (or roughly 2/3) of the cases will have height between 165 and 175, 95% between 160 and 180 and almost all (99.3%) of the cases between 155 and 185 cm.

And in turn if we are choosing a case randomly from the 100 cases, the probability of getting a case of height between 165 and 175 is 68%, so it is common to find a case in this range, and it is easier to find a case of height between 160 and 180 because the probability is 95%. But it is rare to find cases taller or shorter, as the probability of such cases will be 5% only (100% - 95% = 5%)

NB. The probability here is determined by the Frequentist method (chapter 2).

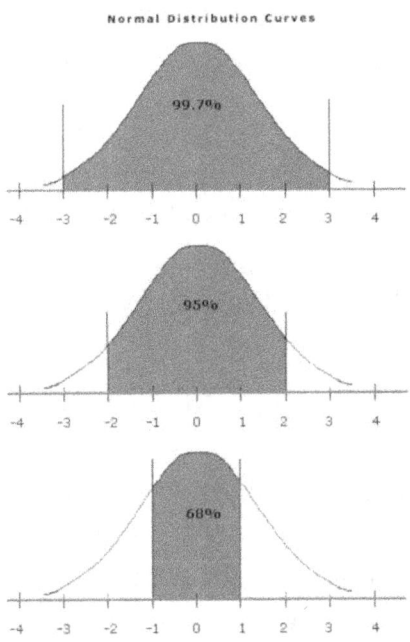

Abnormal distribution

Normal distribution can suffer from some deviations from the previous properties. In this case it is not called abnormal distribution by the way. This deviation may be either due to the nature of the variable we measure itself or due to sampling error.

The variable may have a distorted distribution by its nature, like when trying to categorize people according to their favorite football team. You will find a lot of El-Ahly (or Parcelona) fans and a lot of El-Zamalek (or Real Madrid) fans, but fewer fans for the rest of football teams. In this case the variable is *Bimodal* by its nature regardless how big your sample was.

The other cause of deviation of the properties of normal distribution is the sampling itself, either the sample size or the method of selection. If you have a very small sample, say of 10 individuals, it is unlikely that you will have the curve with prefect normal shape when you plot it, although the variable you measure is normally distributed by nature (like the heights of people).

Another cause is your sampling methodology itself. You can measure the heights of 100 young people of the same age, but without the probable randomization. So you selected them from sports team as it is easier to you to find young people gathered in the same place, if you selected basketball team within your sample, you will notice that the sample mean is deviated towards higher heights, and the curve does not look *normal* at all.

Proper sample size and randomization (selecting your candidates or cases randomly) are 2 crucial conditions to get a normally distributed sample.

Skew

Skew was discussed in detail in chapter 4.

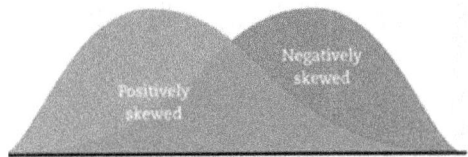

It is important to determine if your data is normally distributed or suffer a skew. This cannot be done by looking at the shape of the curve alone. SPSS software offers a number that represent the amount of skew in the data set (this will be discussed in the SPSS maps part of this book). According the following table you can decide if you are going to neglect the skew and deal with your data as normal distribution or the amount of skew rendered the data into a non-parametric data.

Skew value = 0	Perfectly normal
Skew -1 to +1	Nearly normal
Skew -2 to +2	Not bad
Skew more or less	Skewed distribution

Kurtosis

Kurtosis refers to another characteristic of the curve of data that can render it non-parametric too (not normally distributed).

It means that the tails of the distribution curve are rather too fat (negative kurtosis) or too thin (positive kurtosis). The tail represent the amount of data in the extremes of the scale. In the negative kurtosis, the tail is 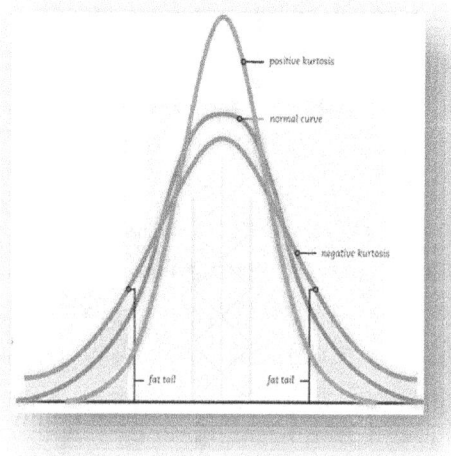 fat, which means that there are more data in the extremes of the scale than usual. In positive kurtosis, the thin tails tells us that the data in the extreme values are scarcer than usual too. In both cases the normal distribution criteria are distorted (specially calculating the probabilities depending on the standard deviation).

Just like skew, kurtosis can be determined using SPSS software according to the following table.

kurtosis value = 0	Perfectly normal
kurtosis -1 to +1	Nearly normal
kurtosis -2 to +2	Not bad
kurtosis more or less	Non-parametric distribution

Normal or not? That is the question

It is important to assume a normal distribution of your data set because this will determine what kind of tests you will use during the rest of your statistical analysis. With non-normally distributed data, there is a whole bundle of statistical tests corresponding to tests for normally distributed data. These tests are called *non-parametric tests.*

For example, to find a correlation between 2 variables. If they are both normally distributed we can use the Pearson test, but if one of them is non-parametric we must use Spearman test (more on this in the next chapters).

Summary

Normal distribution curve

- *Bell shaped*
- *Symmetric* about mean
- *Unimodal*
- *Continuous* distribution
- *Never touches* horizontal axis

Probability of normal distribution

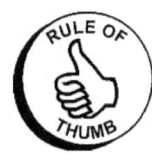

68%   95%   99%

between 1 SD   between 2 SD   between 3 SD

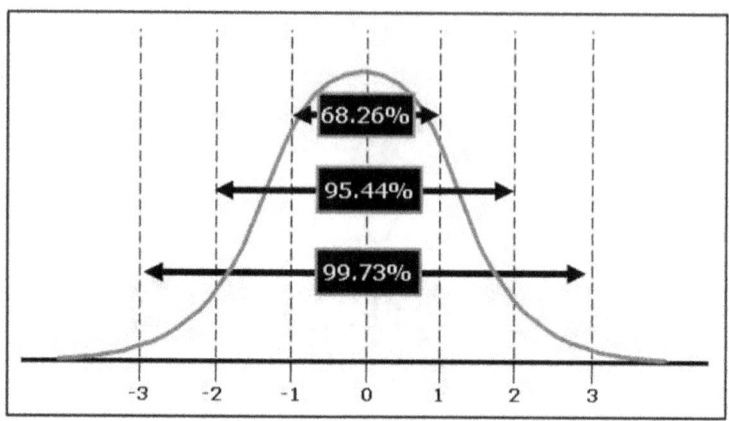

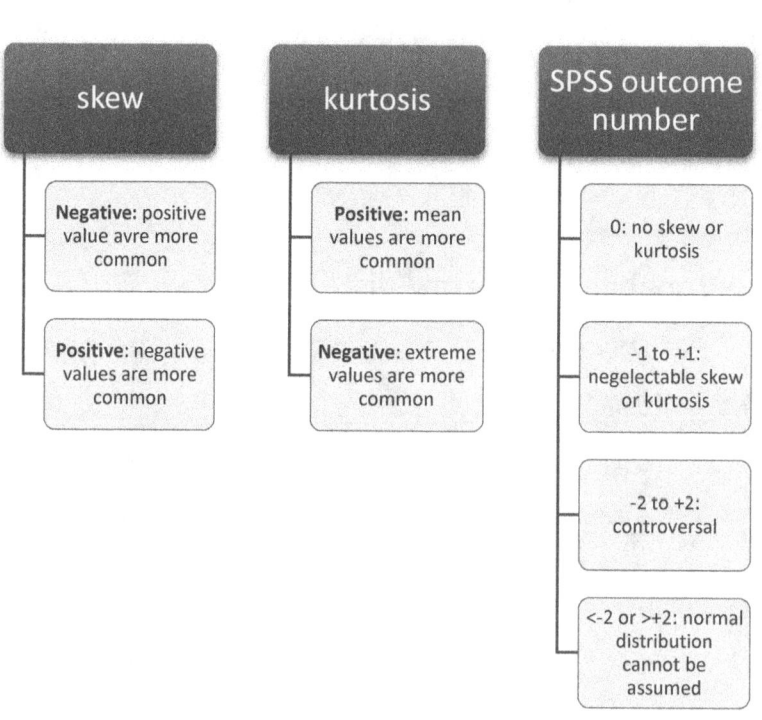

skew

Negative: positive value avre more common

Positive: negative values are more common

kurtosis

Positive: mean values are more common

Negative: extreme values are more common

SPSS outcome number

0: no skew or kurtosis

-1 to +1: negelectable skew or kurtosis

-2 to +2: controversal

<-2 or >+2: normal distribution cannot be assumed

Attention!!

Now you finished the basics and the descriptive methods.

You are about to enter a very powerful zone:

Inferential statistics

Methods explained in the following chapters are so powerful that –if used properly- can enable you to know facts about the entire world population by examining a sample in your local community.

Use them wisely.

Do not cross this page until the previous knowledge is thoroughly understood!

Chapter 6: Confidence Intervals

Learning objectives:

- Sample vs. sampling distribution
- Predicting the parameter through the central limit theorem
- Accuracy vs. precision

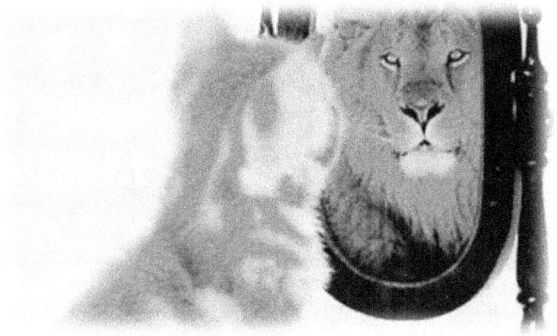

The general idea

The ultimate goal of research is to generalize results of a sample to the entire population. As we discussed before, the sample has statistics (the mean of heights for example) that we try to proof that it is equal to the parameter of the population (the mean of heights of all people). The parameter is unknown as the only way to know it for sure is to measure the heights of the human race and divide its sum by 7 billion (according to the world population watch). But since this is not applicable, our best shot is the sample statistic.

In fact we cannot just assume that our sample's mean equals the population parameter. Simply because if another researcher gathered another sample (even with exactly the same sampling methodology), he will get another value for his sample mean (statistics). Which one of us has the real population parameter? No one can tell.

The solution for this problem is possible through the concept of *confidence intervals (C.I)*. Instead of trying to get the parameter itself, we will get an interval (or a range) in which we can claim confidently that the parameter is somewhere within.

In order to understand the concept of confidence intervals we must go through sample vs. sampling distribution, standard error and central limit theorem. This chapter is the heart of the statistical theory. Grab a cup of coffee and turn the page.

Sample distribution vs. Sampling distribution

Let's start from the top.

➢ We wanted to know the average (mean) height of the human race (the parameter).
➢ We took a sample of 100 person and measured their heights.
➢ Each value of the measure of the height of the 100 persons is a datum, they all together form the sample distribution.
➢ The mean of this sample was 173 cm.
➢ Another group of researchers took another sample of another 100 persons, the mean height in their sample was 171 cm.
➢ This research became popular, and another 2 groups repeated it. The means was 173.5 and 169 cm.

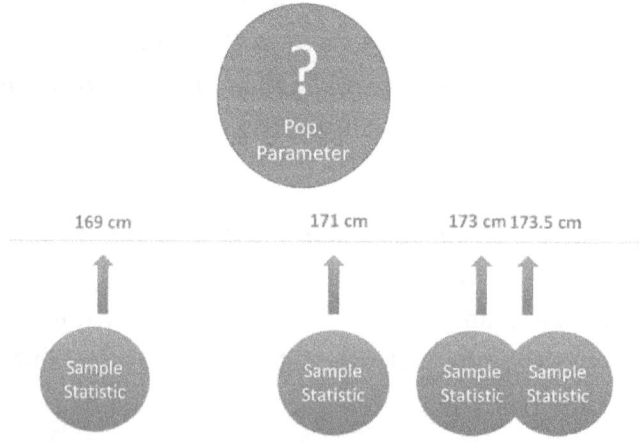

➢ Now we have 4 means but no parameter yet.

- Let's now suppose that we have the means of 100 research groups done for 100 different sample.
- We will construct a new data set, its data points are not the measurements of the cases, but instead it is the means of each sample. This is what is called *sampling distribution.*
- The mean of all the means *(mean of the sampling distribution)* will be the real parameter.

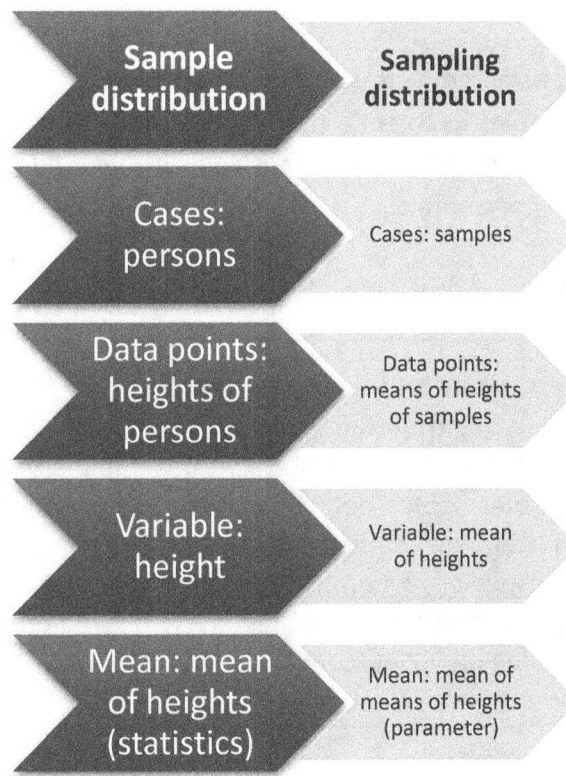

Central limit theorem

Till now we managed to guess the population parameter from the mean of sampling distribution. But this method has its drawbacks. First of all it is unrealistic, as in real life situations we have only one sample not many samples to construct a sampling distribution. The second issue that is gives us a single value that could be not accurate, we need a method to give us an interval instead in which the parameter lies within.

The central limit theorem can fix both of these problems. It enables us to get a sampling distribution from a single sample and in the same time it gives us a confidence interval for the parameter.

Central limit theorem

The sampling distribution of the sampling means approaches <u>a normal distribution</u> as the sample size gets larger, regardless of the shape of the population distribution. So the sample means will be normally distributed <u>(especially when the sample is above 30)</u> if the population is positively skewed, negatively skewed or even binomial (having only 2 outcomes).

In the last chapter we discussed the concept of sample distribution, it can be normally distributed or suffer a degree of skew or kurtosis. But the central limit theorem tells us that the sampling distribution is always *normal* if we extracted it from a sample of size larger than 30 cases.

How can we extract it?

This can be done by constructing the curve of normal distribution.

The curve is formed from a mean in the center and standard deviations (1st, 2nd and 3rd) on the horizontal axis. These SDs mark the amount of data under the curve (68%, 95% and 99% respectively).

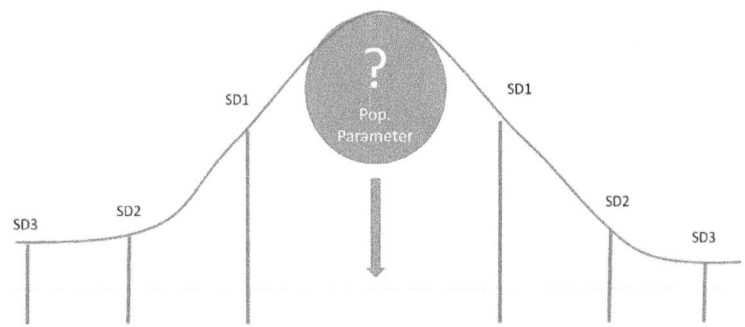

We will not guess the mean as it is the parameter, we want to get it as an interval, but we can put our sample mean in the center of the curve to build the interval around it. We will guess only the SD to construct the curve. This can be done by finding the *Standard error.*

The standard error (SE) is our best guess for the standard deviation of the sampling distribution. It equals the

$$SE = SD/\sqrt{n}$$

division of the SD of our sample by the square root of sample size (number of cases of our sample = n).

The standard error of the sampling distribution is the equivalent to the standard deviation in the sample distribution. It simply means the margin of error of the sampling distribution to define the parameter. The same rules of probability apply here as in sample distribution. The probability of finding the mean (parameter) between the values of the first standard errors (-1 SE & +1 SE) is 68%, between the second SE (-2 SE & +2 SE) is 95% and the third SE (-3 SE & +3 SE) is 99.3%.

In other words, we can say that we are sure by 95% that the parameter lies between the second SE. this is called the 95% confidence interval.

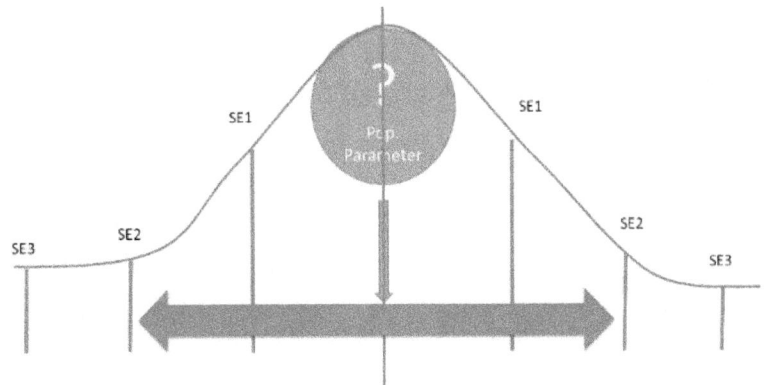

Between the 2nd positive and negative SE lies the 95% confidence interval of the mean.

For example:

- ➤ We wanted to know the average (mean) height of the human race (the parameter).
- ➤ We took a sample of 100 person and measured their heights.
- ➤ Each height of the 100 measures is a datum, they all together form the sample distribution.
- ➤ The mean of this sample was 173 cm and the SD was 10.
- ➤ We calculate the SE = 10/√100 = 1
- ➤ The sampling distribution curve will be as follows:

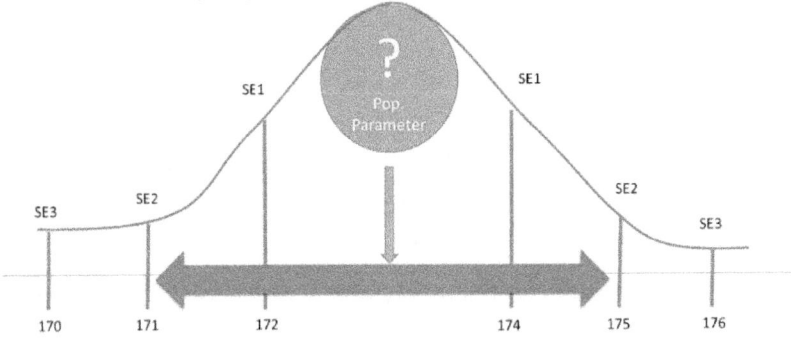

➢ The 95% Confidence interval (95% C. I.) = -2 SE to + 2 SE

➢ 95% C. I. = 171 – 175

➢ We are sure by 95% that the parameter (the average height of the human race) is somewhere between 171 cm and 175 cm.

Accuracy vs. Precision

Accuracy: the ability of the confidence interval to hit the real parameter.

Precision: the ability of the confidence interval to precisely define the parameter within a narrow range.

If we assumed that the parameter of the height of the human race lies within the 95% C.I. 130 to 220 cm. we are now accurate, as the parameter must be within this range. But we are not precise as we gave a very wide range, which although almost cannot miss the parameter, it is useless as it cannot be used in clinical practice. On the other hand, if we gave a precise range from 171 to 171.5 cm. It is very useful as it almost defined the parameter in a single value, but it is not very accurate, as the parameter can be slightly higher or lower than this value.

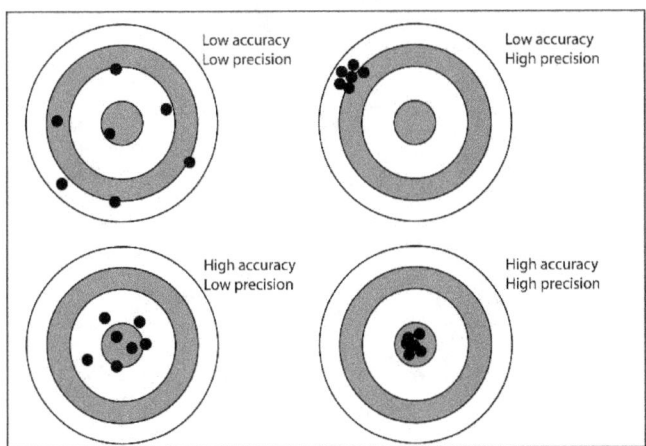

- To increase accuracy: take a wide Confidence interval. Most studies accept the 95% C.I. but you can use a wider range as the 99% C.I. In this case you will use the interval between -3 SE and +3 SE.

- To increase precision: decrease the value SE to make the confidence interval narrower. This can be done by either decrease the SD or increase the sample size (n). And since the SD cannot be manipulated because it is extracted from the data. The only way to increase precision is to increase the sample size, which in turn gives you a lower values of SE, and a narrower (more precise) C. I.

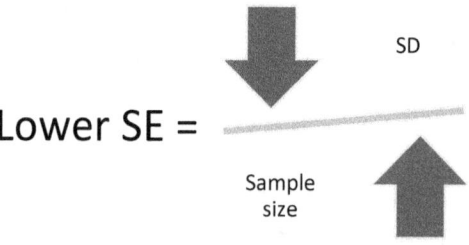

Lower SE = $\dfrac{\text{SD}}{\text{Sample size}}$

Summary

Sample distribution	Sampling distribution
• Of a certain variable • Mean is a statistic	• Of means of a certain variable • Mean is the parameter

Variables – Means of variable	Mean – Parameter (population mean)	SD – Standard error

Central limit theorem	Confidence interval
• Sampling distribution have normal distrbution around the mean (parameter)	• Where we are 95% sure to find the mean (parameter)

Accuracy Vs. Precision

• Increase sample size to adjust percison

The sample mean is the best possible center point estimate of the C.I.

2 is a constant that depends on the level of confidence. For 95% we put to and for 99% we put 3.

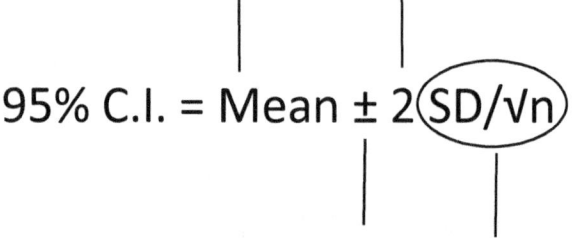

$$95\% \text{ C.I.} = \text{Mean} \pm 2(SD/\sqrt{n})$$

± Sign creates the interval. Define its lower and upper margins by subtracting the following value from and add it to the mean.

This is the margin of error, also known as the standard error of the mean. It depends on the SD and the sample size.

Chapter 7: Null Hypothesis Significance Testing

Learning objectives:

- Steps of the scientific method
- Null vs. alternative hypothesis
- Steps of the null hypothesis judging
- P value and alpha level
- Errors of null hypothesis significance testing; type I & II errors

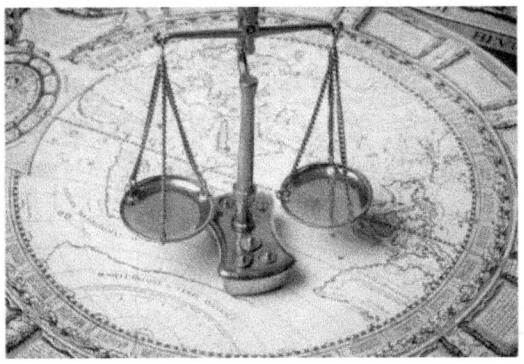

The scientific method

I remember studying the menstrual cycle 4 times during my entire study (this apply to the Egyptian educational system only): in the 3rd preparatory grade, 2nd secondary grade, 2nd year of medical school in physiology and finally 6th year in medical school in gynecology. With every time knew aspects were discussed and a wider vision acquired.

But I blame the educational system for teaching me the scientific method of thinking once throughout my education in the 4th grade of primary school. It is really unfair to teach such young minds the foundation of our modern science once and for all.

The scientific method of thinking consists of certain steps that should be followed respectively in order to reach a scientific solution of any given problem, from gravity and movement of planets to the effect of medications on the body physiology. Even to decide the best way to drive to work or the explanation behind your repeated internet connection problems, you can use the scientific method.

These steps can be defined as following:

- **Step 1: define the problem**

State your problem in clear, unambiguous words in the form of a question. *What is the fastest way to drive to work?*

- **Step 2: state the hypothesizes**

Think of possible solutions for your problem. Think of as many as you can either inside or outside the box. *It is faster* to drive through way A (your usual way). It is faster to drive through way B (a new way you want to try).

- **Step 3: examine the hypothesizes**

Put an indicator to judge if the hypothesis fulfill your purpose or not. *The way that takes the shortest time on a non-stop trip is considered faster.*

- **Step 4: carry out an experiment/research**

Design an experiment or a research policy to decide which hypothesis is true. *I will drive to work through way A and register the time, then on the same day next week and at the same hour I will drive through way B and register the time.*

Note that while designing the experiment/research you should take care of certain points such as:

Applicability: the experiment is easily applied without so much resources needed. *It is just a drive to work with a stopwatch.*

Isolation of confounders: confounders are factors that can affect the result of your research giving you false results in favor of either hypothesizes. *For example if you tried way A on Saturday at 8 am and way B on Friday at 10 am, way B will seem much faster even in fact it was not because you are trying it on the weekend. Here the rush hours are confounders that you failed to isolate. So you must try both ways on exactly the same conditions: the same day of the week, the same hour and the same driver.*

- **Step 5: reach a conclusion**

After getting your results, compare it to find the appropriate answer to your question. *If way A takes 9 minutes and way B takes 12 minutes, then the answer to your question is that: way A is the fastest way to drive to work.*

The Null hypothesis vs. the alternative Hypothesis

While going through the scientific method you need to examine each hypothesis separately (in step 3). Here you should use the concept of null hypothesis.

Null means nothing, nonexistent, empty or non-effective.

The null hypothesis is the hypothesis that the factor we are examining has no effect. This is the start point of any research, that the hypothesis we are testing is not effective. The idea behind this concept is: in the natural world, the basal condition of any 2 factors that they are isolated, unrelated and do not affect each other. If you proved that this fact is wrong, then there is a relation between these 2 factors. This is the *alternative hypothesis.*

For example:

Is there a relation between the following factors (medications) and the heart rate?

- Propranolol[4]
- Paracetamol[5]

First we would assume that we know nothing about both drugs. So it is wise to assume that both of them do not affect the heart rate till proven otherwise.

Our null hypothesis (denoted as H_0) will be:

---

[4] Generalized beta blocker
[5] Antipyretic

- H_{01}: propranolol does not affect heart rate.
- H_{02}: paracetamol does not affect heart rate.

If we managed to prove any of the above false, this will prove that the opposite (the alternative hypothesis, denoted as: H_a) is true. So the H_a must be the exact opposite of the H_0.

- H_{a1}: propranolol affects the heart rate.
- H_{a2}: paracetamol affects the heart rate.

Null hypothesis and Alternative hypothesis can NEVER co-exist in the same universe, because they are the exact opposite of each other. Rejecting one of them alter the other accepted without the need of further evidence.

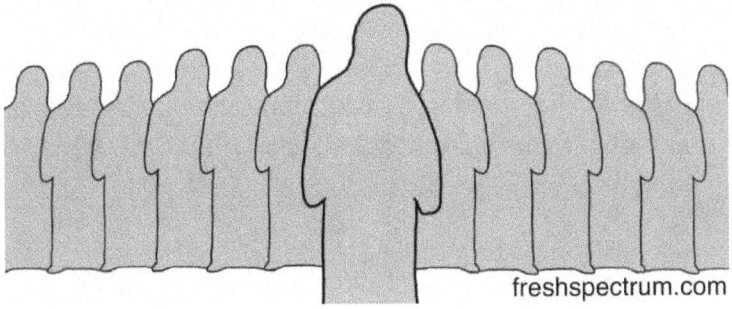

I am what is
The default, the status quo
I am already accepted, can only be rejected
The burden of proof is on the alternative

I am the null hypothesis

freshspectrum.com

The Null hypothesis significance testing process

Now carry out an experiment/research while assuming that H_{01} is true. After you get the final results, decide the following: what is the probability of getting this results while the H_{01} is true. If the probability is high, this means that the null hypothesis is true and cannot be rejected. So the alternative hypothesis is false. If the probability is low, then the null hypothesis is false and can be rejected. Then the alternative hypothesis is true without the need of any further proof.

Let's apply the previous methodology in more depth. We are now examining H_{a1}: propranolol affects the heart rate.

Step 1: gather a suitable sample, say 100 healthy persons. Measure their pulse (variable: pulse1 or p1) – give them propranolol – measure their pulse again (variable: pulse2 or p2).

Step 2: the variable p1 can predict the parameter of the mean of the normal pulse. P1 mean = 80 b/m, SD = 10 b/m, number of cases n = 100.

$SE = SD/\sqrt{n} = 10/\sqrt{100} = 1$

The 95% C. I. for the parameter of normal pulse mean is from -2 SE of the mean to +2 SE of the mean = 78 – 82 b/m.

I.e. we are sure by 95% that the mean of the normal pulse of the population is between 78 and 82 b/m.

Step 3: the variable p2 can predict the parameter of the mean of the pulse after propranolol intake. P2 mean = 60 b/m, SD = 10 b/m.

Step 4: now let's assume that the null hypothesis is true (H_{01}: propranolol does not affect heart rate.) This means that the pulse after propranolol intake (p2) will be the same as the parameter of normal pulse (p1).

Step 5: let's now draw the probability curve of the sampling distribution. And calculate the probability of getting a pulse of 60 b/m.

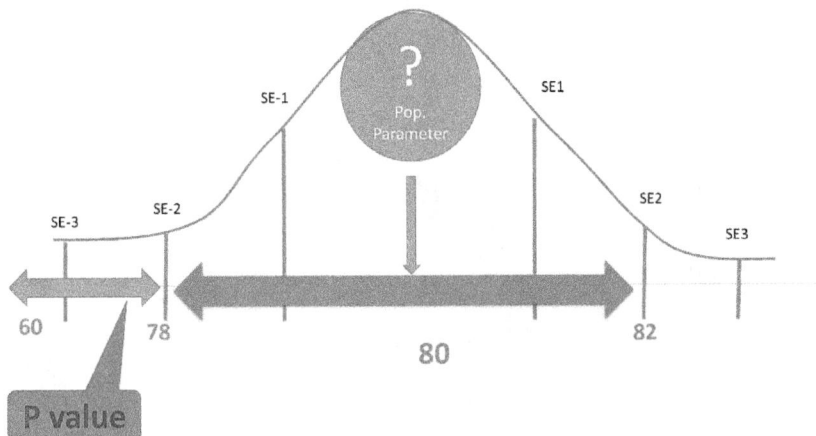

✓ The whole area under the curve = the probability of getting any value of pulse parameter = 100% or 1.

✓ The probability of the normal pulse between 78 and 82 = 95% or 0.95.

✓ The probability of the parameter being less than 78 or greater than 82 = 5% or 0.05.

✓ The probability of being less than 78 only is 5%/2 = 2.5% or 0.025, and the same for greater than 82 only.

✓ The probability of the normal parameter being 60 is much less than 2.5%. Say 1% or 0.01. *This is called the p value.*

P value (Significance): *The probability of getting a certain result or more extreme yet the null hypothesis is true.*

In other words, it is the probability of getting a parameter of 60 b/m after propranolol, yet the null hypothesis which says that there is no effect is true. I.e. pulse after propranolol (p2) = normal pulse (p1).

We agreed that if this probability or p value is low we will reject the null hypothesis because it will be very unlikely to be true.

But how can we decide if the p value is low or not?

This is done by the alpha (α) level.

Alpha (α) level: It is a level of probability decided before the research begin, below which the p value will be considered very low or insignificant. It is usually 0.05, but some researches require a lower level of 0.01.

In our research we decided that α level = 0.05. We found that the p value for pulse after propranolol (p2 = 60 b/m) and still equal to the normal pulse that we calculated a 95% C. I. for it. This p value was 0.01. So we can consider it too low, and the H_{01} too unlikely.

Null hypothesis rejected.

Alternative Hypothesis accepted.

Conclusion: propranolol affects the heart rate.

The possible outcomes Null hypothesis significance testing

If the null hypothesis was false and we rjected it, then we did a good job. Also if the null hypothesis was true and we retained it (and rejected the alternative hypothesis), then we did a good job too.

But what if an error occurred during our calculations?

There are possible types of errors:

i.   Rejecting a true null hypothesis: **Type I error.**

ii.   Retaining a false null hypothesis: **Type II error.**

Type I error represents a false alarm. Your data was really insignificant, but you said that there is a significant effect. While in type II error, you had a significant data but you failed to prove its significant throught the statistical methods. This is like a miss shoot that failed to hit the target.

At the end of this chapter you must know that: the main idea of null hypothesis significance testing applies to the whole infrential statistical methods. When you want to make any infrence about the population, whatever the effect you are assessing is, assume that there is no effect, then try to reject this hypothesis by proofing that it is very unlikely to have your results when there is no effect (i.e. when the null hypothesis is true).

This effect can be: difference of means, correlation between 2 variables or survival ananlysis etc.. we will discuss the correlation between 2 variables in the next chapter, and the rest of infrential methods are byeond the scope of this book. But now at least you can understand the meaning of the p value associated with any statistical test. And on this base, you can easily understand any infrential method.

Summary

Steps of the scientific method

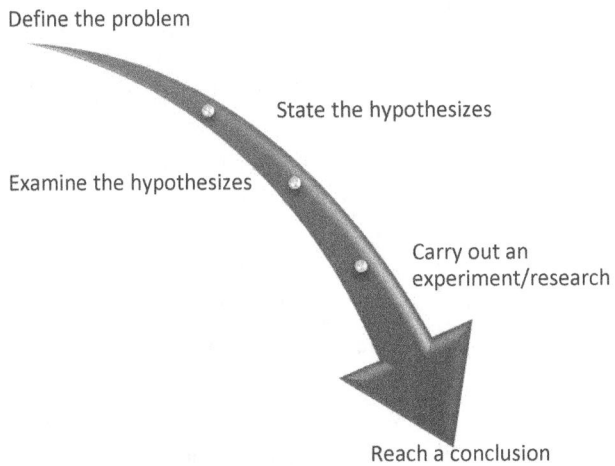

Define the problem

State the hypothesizes

Examine the hypothesizes

Carry out an
experiment/research

Reach a conclusion

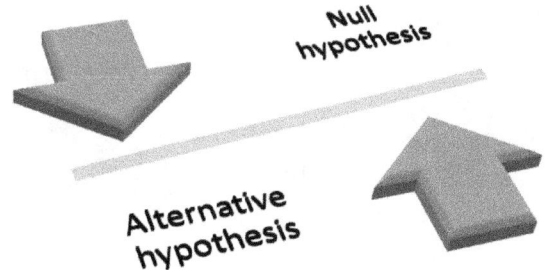

Null
hypothesis

Alternative
hypothesis

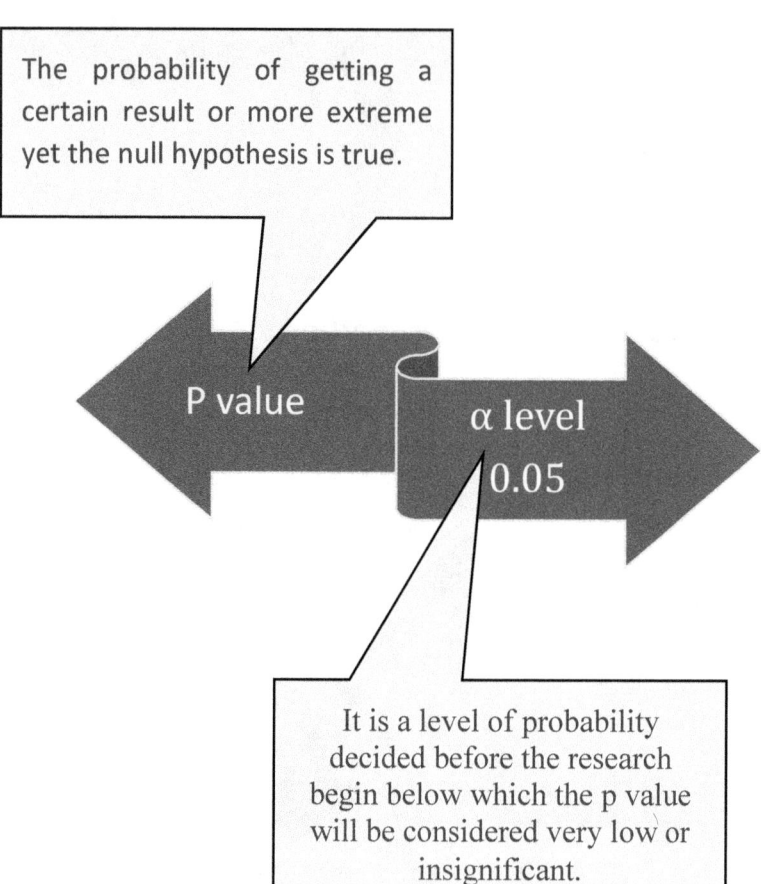

The probability of getting a certain result or more extreme yet the null hypothesis is true.

P value

α level
0.05

It is a level of probability decided before the research begin below which the p value will be considered very low or insignificant.

	Retain H_0	Reject H_0
H_0 true	Correct	Type I error (false alarm)
H_0 false	Type II error (a miss)	Correct

Chapter 8: Correlation

Learning objectives:

- Linear correlation
- Scatter plot graph
- Correlation coefficient; Pearson's & Spearman's
- Causation and the concept of confounders

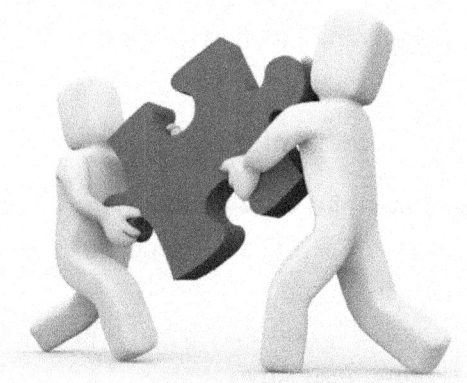

The idea of correlation depends on finding a relation between 2 variables. This relation could be directly proportional; when one variable increases, the other increases too, or inversely proportional; when one decreases the other increases.

Directly proportional relations are called: "positive correlation", while inversely proportional relations are called: "negative correlation".

The idea of Null hypothesis significance testing applies to the concept of correlation. The H_0 usually assumes that there is no relation between the 2 variables. Then it can be rejected by examining the data – as we will describe in this chapter.

The steps of correlational analysis are as follows:

1. Define the 2 variables you want to investigate.
2. Define the null and alternative hypothesizes.
3. Build a scatter plot graph.
4. Calculate the correlation coefficient and its p value.
5. Reject or retain the null hypothesis.

Scatter plot – Graphical illustration

The scatter plot is the best way to illustrate correlation between 2 variables. On the horizontal axis a variable is plotted and the other is plotted on the vertical axis. The dots represents the values of each case on both scales (variables). The following graph represent the scatter plot for the variables weight and height.

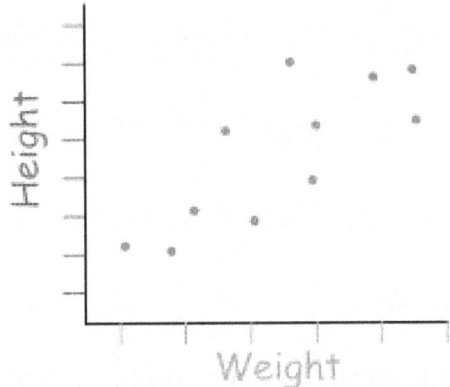

The scatter plot can tell you the following information:

- Is there a relation or not?
- What is its type (positive or negative?)
- Is it linear or curvilinear?
- Is it a strong relation or a weak one?

So it is wise to build the scatter plot as a second step after defining your variables of interest. This enables you to know a lot of information about the relation before starting a deeper analysis.

Possible outcomes of the scatter-plot:

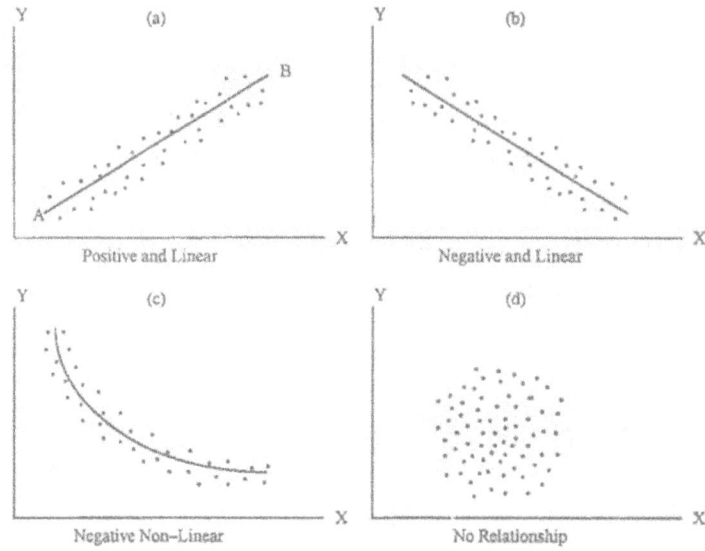

1- **Relation or not?**

In the above figure, there is a relation between the variables X & Y in graphs: a, b and c. While in graph d there is no relation. In the graphs that represent a relation, you can find a certain pattern of the dots (cases) that looks more or less like a line. While in graph d you can see that the dots are scattered randomly in the middle of the graph, indicating the absence of relation.

The pattern is more evident when you examine each dot alone. You will find that in graph a for example that dots that represent lower values of the X scale (to the left) also represent lower values on Y scale (below). And higher values of X (to the Right) have higher values for Y (above). And the opposite for graphs b & c where higher Xs means Lower Ys.

But in graph d the pattern is lost, where you can find dots with high values of X and low values of Y, and others with high values on both scales (X & Y) and so on.

2- Positive or negative?

When the dots for and increasing line (like: /) it means that values on both scales increases and decreases together. If the line is in the opposite direction (like: \), then when X increases Y decreases and vice versa.

So a line /: denotes a positive relation (graph a), and a line \: denotes a negative relation (graph b & c).

3- Linear or curvilinear?

Graphs a & b represent linear relations, where the rate of change of both values is constant for all data points or cases. I.e. values of X increase by the same value with increasing value of Y. While in graph c the curve (not line) of dots represents a changing rate of change. I.e. sometimes values of X increase a little bit or much more with the same increase of value of Y.

4- Strong or weak?

The strength of the correlation is better demonstrated by the correlation coefficient (discussed later), but the scatter plot graph gives a hint about the strength.

A correlation is considered strong if each case shows equal change in both variables together. That is not always the situation, in real life situation there is always variations in the changes occurring in different cases.

The following graphs show variable strengths of positive correlations, varying from a weak relation to a perfect correlation which is the strongest form.

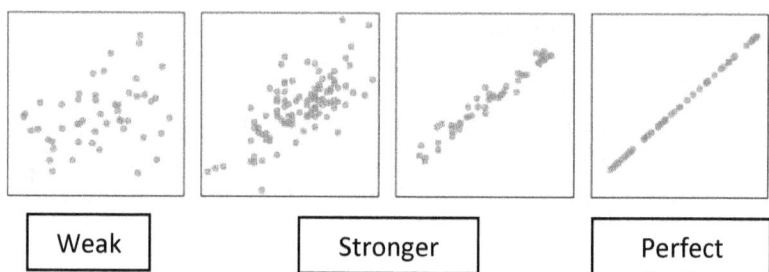

Notice that with the increase of the strength, the dots are arranged in a form of a narrower line, till the perfect form in which a perfect line appears.

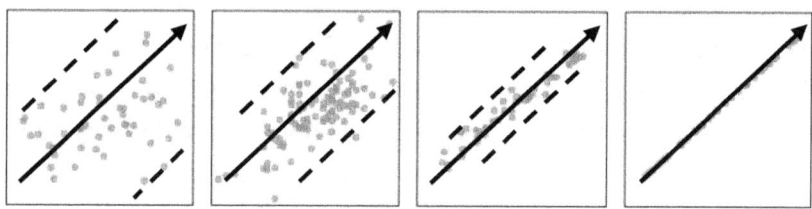

The correlation coefficient[6]

The correlation coefficient (denoted as: r) is a numerical representation of the strength of the correlation.

The (ugly) equation used to calculate this number is as follows:

$$r = \frac{\sum xy}{\sqrt{\sum x^2 \sum y^2}}$$

Where did this come from? It is the ratio between the degree of variation of x and y together (covariance) and the degree of x and y variation independently (variance x and y)

The good news that you do not really need to memorize this equation or even know how it is calculated, because computer software do it in milliseconds. The important part is to understand its outcome and how can you interpret it.

The meaning of this equation that r represents correlation in the following way.

✓ Each of X & Y varies alone (variance in descriptive statistics).
✓ X and Y varies together due to their mutual effect.

---

[6] In this chapter we will discuss linear correlation only. Although there are statistical methods to evaluate non-linear correlation, but they are far advanced in respect to the level of this book.

✓ How much of "varies together" is due to the effect of them on each other and how much is due to their natural variance independently?

This is a ratio. As any ratio it is a number between 0 and 1, where 0 means absence of any relation or in other words, 0 means that all the change in either X or Y is due to the independent variance of each variable and 0% is due to their effect on each other.

Also 1 means that there is a perfect correlation between X & Y, or in other words, 1 means that none of the change in either X or Y is due to the independent variance of each variable and 100% is due to their effect on each other.

Any decimal in between represents the percentage of the change due to the mutual effect in relation to the independent change. For example if r = 0.67, then 67% of the change in variable X is due to variable Y and the remaining change (100 − 67 = 33%) is due to variance of X alone.

To denote the positive nature of the correlation the coefficient takes + or − sign, rendering it as a number between -1 and +1.

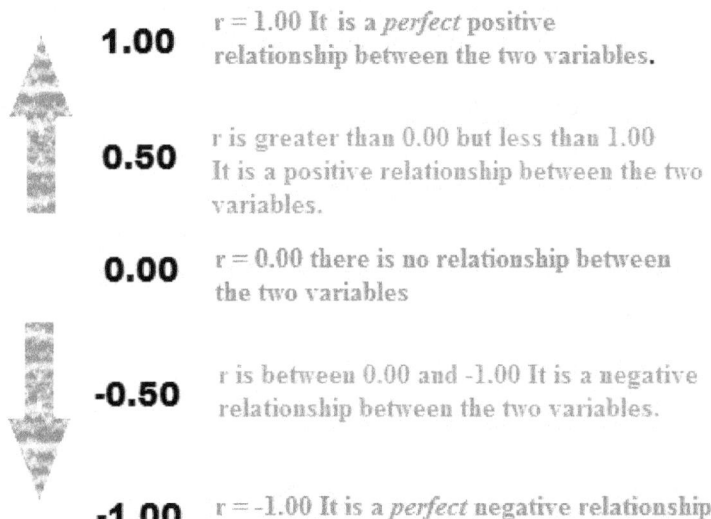

r = 1.00 It is a *perfect* positive relationship between the two variables.

r is greater than 0.00 but less than 1.00 It is a positive relationship between the two variables.

r = 0.00 there is no relationship between the two variables

r is between 0.00 and -1.00 It is a negative relationship between the two variables.

r = -1.00 It is a *perfect* negative relationship between the two variables.

Now we can combine the value of r and the shape of the scatter plot to understand the nature of the correlation in the following figure.

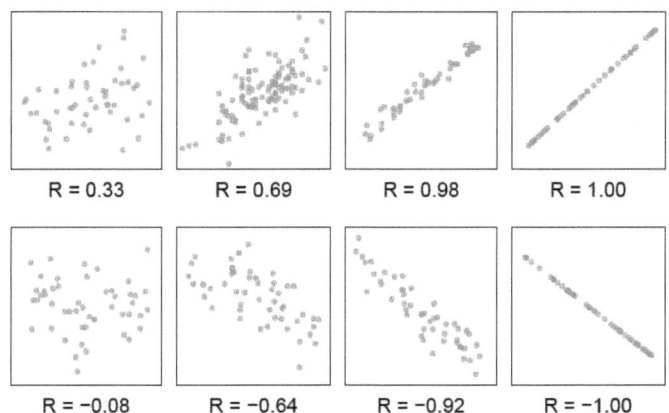

After calculating the value of r, the software will give you another important value; which is the p value. As we said before: the p value is the probability of getting a data in which the r of the 2 factors = 0.67 for instance, and yet the null hypothesis is true (there is no correlation).

In other words, the p value is the probability of the r = 0.67 being due to chance alone not due to correlation. If the p value is very low (below α level – usually 0.05) then it is unlikely that the r is only due to chance. Reject the H_0, accept the H_a and enjoy your statistically significant correlation. And vice versa of course.

The choice of correlation coefficient

As we said earlier in chapter 4 (normal distribution). There is usually statistical test for normally distributed continuous (or scale) variables, and a non-parametric equivalent test for ordinal variables and/or non-normally distributed scale variables.

There are 2 main types of correlation coefficients that can both be calculated by computer software:

① **Pearson (r)** is between 2 continuous variables (normally distributed).

② **Spearman** between 2 ordinal variables or 2 continuous (not normally distributed variables).

The conditions that must be established to use the Pearson correlation is stated below, otherwise use the Spearman correlation test.

Conditions for Pearson correlation coefficient:

1- **2 contentious variables**

2- **X , Y have normal distribution**

3- **Linear relationship between X, Y** Not curvilinear (Examine a scatterplot to ensure this)

N.B: *Spearman is not used for curvilinear correlation.*

Confounders and causation

Be careful when using correlation!

While it looks simple enough to use correlation, and looks tempting to plot variables against each other searching for hidden relations. Be careful of what you wish for. Random choice of variables can turn your research into a joke. Like the following example:

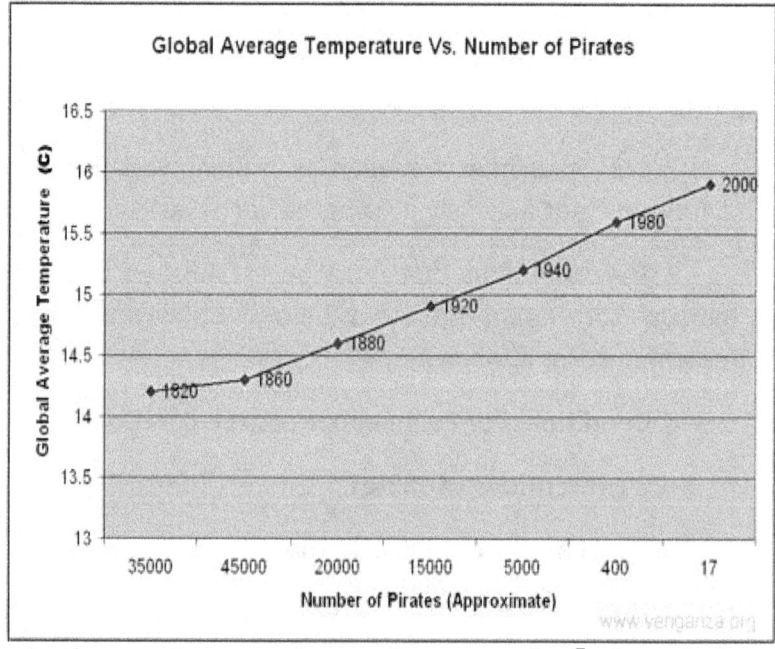

In the previous graph, a naïve researcher[7] plotted the global average temperature (vertical axis) against the number of pirates (horizontal axis). Surprisingly, he found a

---

[7] Mostly a big fan of "Pirates of the Caribbean" and "The day after tomorrow" too.

strong negative correlation[8]. There are a whole punch of weird explanation of the fact that the decrease in the number of pirates led to global warming. Try to think of some!

But how did this happened? Certainly there is an explanation other than that the act of piracy protects the Earth climate. The answer to this question is simply: *the confounder.*

As discussed before, a confounder is a factor that is not inspected during the research although it is the real cause behind the noticed effect.

The confounder here is the development of major countries in the industrial era. The developed countries developed bigger economies then larger armies that could manage to cut down the pirates' population. Meanwhile, bigger economies came with bigger factories and more green-house effect producing products, which led to the increase in the mean global temperature.

---

[8] Notice that the horizontal axis variable is plotted in descending order, this reversed the shape of negative relation to the line / instead of the usual \ line.

Bottom line: correlation does not imply causation. High quality research that take in count every possible confounder should be done first to assume causation based on correlation. So, do not get too excited when you found a correlation.

Summary

The steps of correlational analysis

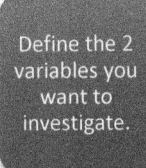

| Define the 2 variables you want to investigate. | Define H_0 and H_a. | Build a scatter plot graph. | Calculate the correlation coefficient and its p value. | Reject or retain the null hypothesis. |

Interpretation of the value of r

Negative r
- inverse correaltion
- a variable ↑ the other ↓

Positive r
- direct correlation
- both variables ↑ or ↓ together

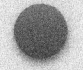

Zero r
- no correlation

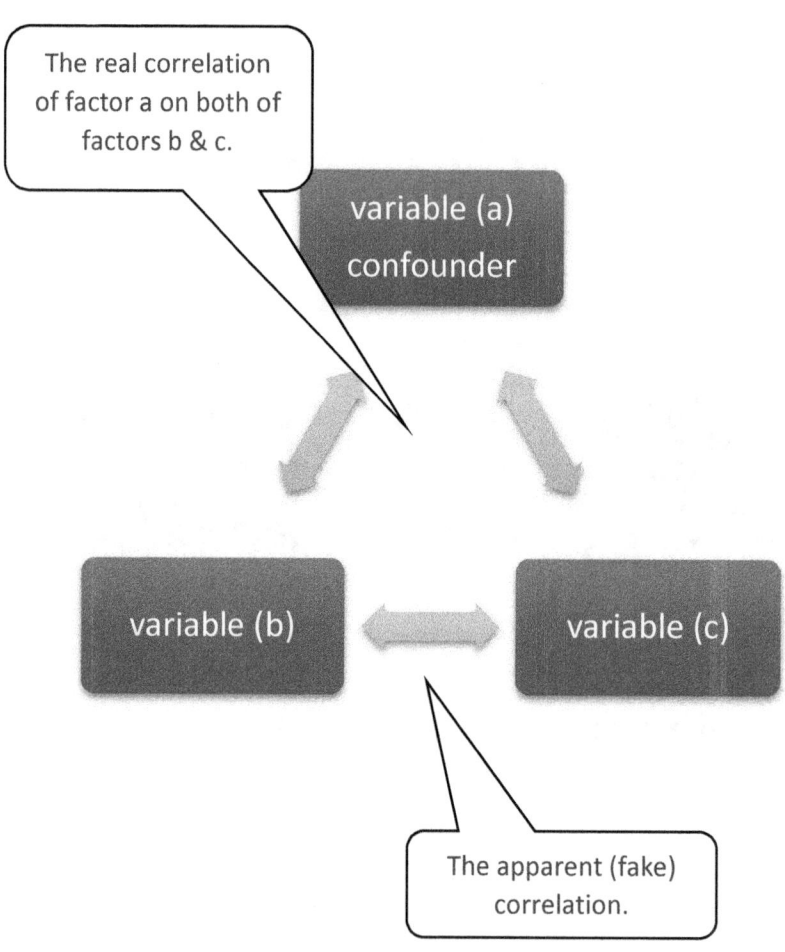

SPSS maps

SPSS maps section is not meant to be used as a stand-alone tool for learning how to use SPSS. I believe that skills like using a software are better transmitted through hands-on training. Yet, you can find this section extremely helpful if you used it as a guide to start your experience with SPSS, a reminder of knowledge you already acquired earlier or any other creative use including absorbing extra oil of the French fries.

Remember, these are maps. A guide through your road. Not a complete manual of the journey.

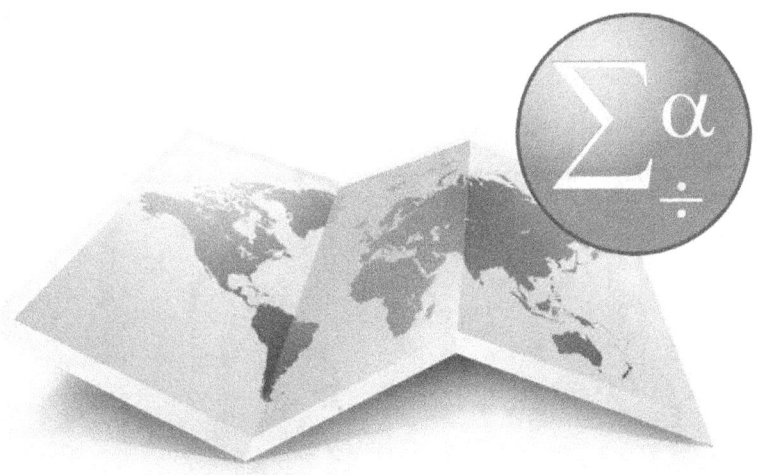

Step 1: prepare your data

Customize your data in the "variable view"

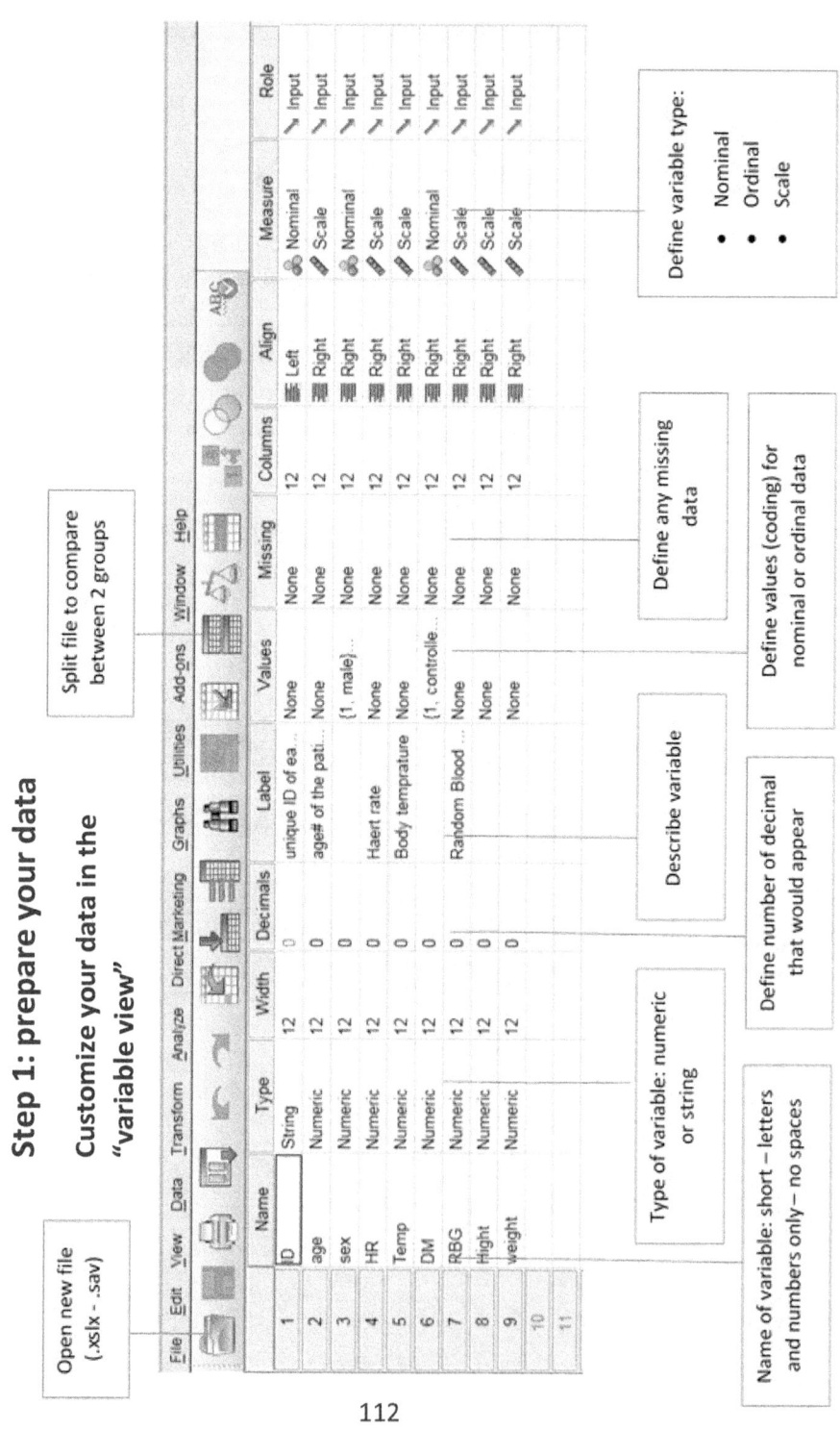

Open new file (.xslx - .sav)

Split file to compare between 2 groups

	Name	Type	Width	Decimals	Label	Values	Missing	Columns	Align	Measure	Role
1	ID	String	12	0	unique ID of ea..	None	None	12	Left	Nominal	Input
2	age	Numeric	12	0	age# of the pati..	None	None	12	Right	Scale	Input
3	sex	Numeric	12	0		{1, male}..	None	12	Right	Nominal	Input
4	HR	Numeric	12	0	Haert rate	None	None	12	Right	Scale	Input
5	Temp	Numeric	12	0	Body temprature	None	None	12	Right	Scale	Input
6	DM	Numeric	12	0		{1, controlle..	None	12	Right	Nominal	Input
7	RBG	Numeric	12	0	Random Blood ..	None	None	12	Right	Scale	Input
8	Hight	Numeric	12	0		None	None	12	Right	Scale	Input
9	weight	Numeric	12	0		None	None	12	Right	Scale	Input
10											
11											

Define variable type:
- Nominal
- Ordinal
- Scale

Define any missing data

Define values (coding) for nominal or ordinal data

Describe variable

Define number of decimal that would appear

Type of variable: numeric or string

Name of variable: short – letters and numbers only– no spaces

112

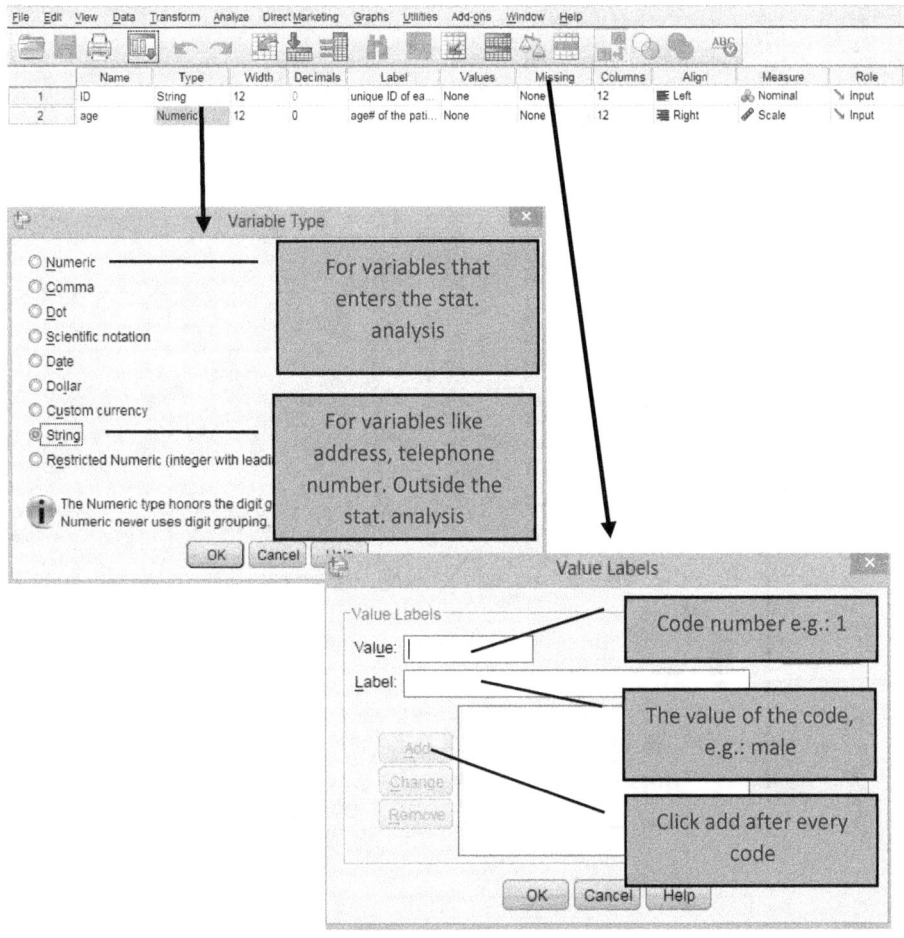

Variable type enables SPSS to distinguish between statistically relevant variables (numeric) and variables used to track the cases e.g. ID, serial numbers etc.

Value labels enable SPSS to handle discrete variables (nominal or ordinal) as numbers, where each number represent a certain value. E.g. variable SEX have the following codes: 1 = male, 2 = female.

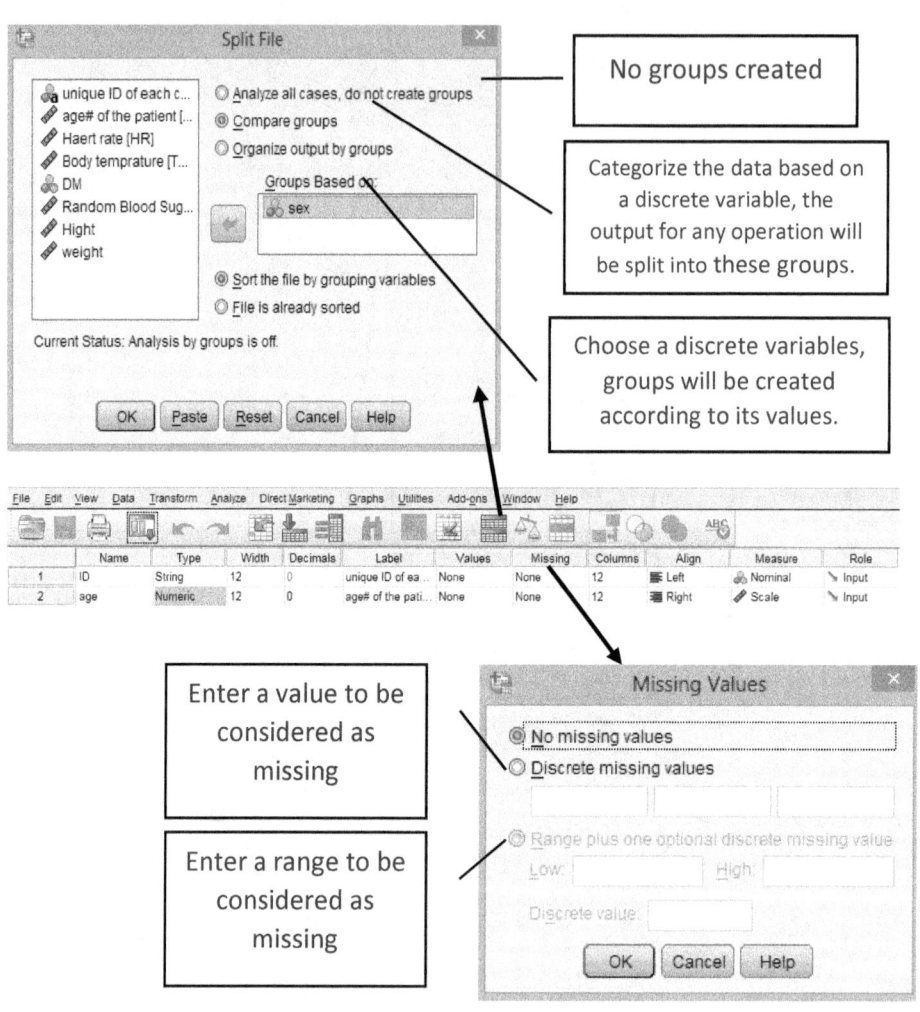

No groups created

Categorize the data based on a discrete variable, the output for any operation will be split into these groups.

Choose a discrete variables, groups will be created according to its values.

Enter a value to be considered as missing

Enter a range to be considered as missing

Missing values could be either absent during data collection or outlier that you want to discard. This enable you to preserve the case while ignoring the missing datum without affecting the sample size.

Step 2: data entry

Enter new data or create variable automatic in "Data View"

Variable (column)

Case (Row)

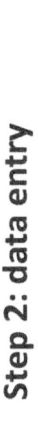

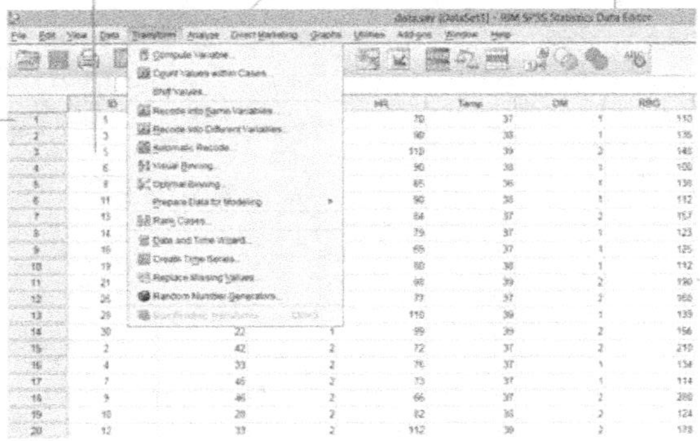

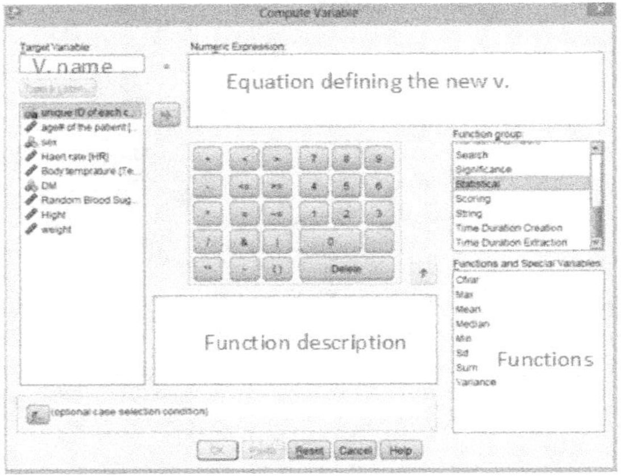

Analyze > Descriptive

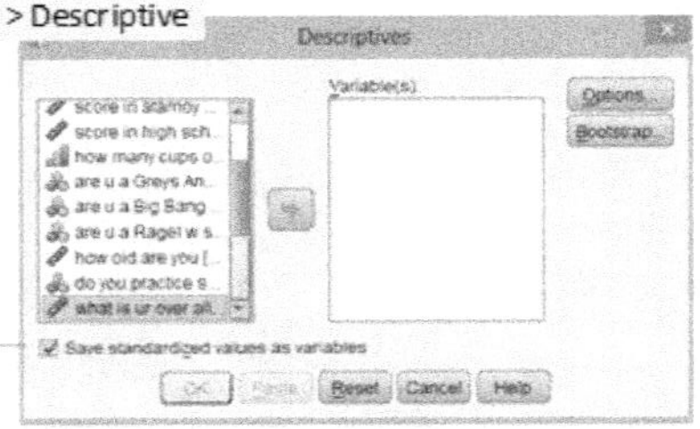

Create new variables with z score

Also check for duplicated cases in Data> define duplicate cases

Step 3: Descriptive Statistics

Perform Descriptive statistics on your data set including: Central tendency, spread, graphs and evaluate normality

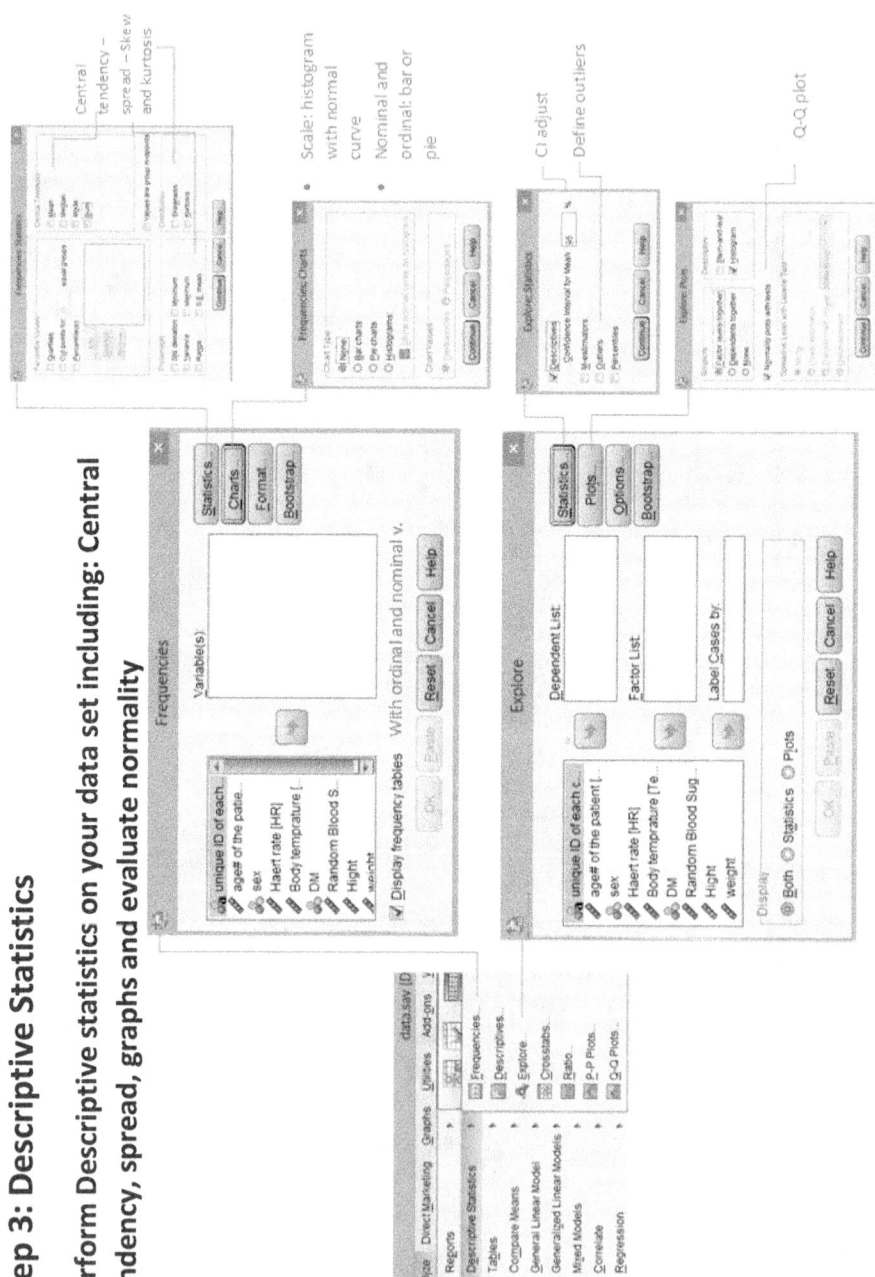

Output of SPSS for frequencies option

Statistics

Haert rate

Variable name		
Number of cases		

N	Valid	30
	Missing	0
Mean		85.43
Std. Error of Mean		2.766
Median		80.50
Mode		90
Std. Deviation		15.151
Variance		229.564
Skewness		.679
Std. Error of Skewness		.427
Kurtosis		-.644
Std. Error of Kurtosis		.833
Range		53
Percentiles	25	72.75
	50	80.50
	75	98.25

Central tendency

Variance measures, skew & kurtosis

Histogram with normal curve

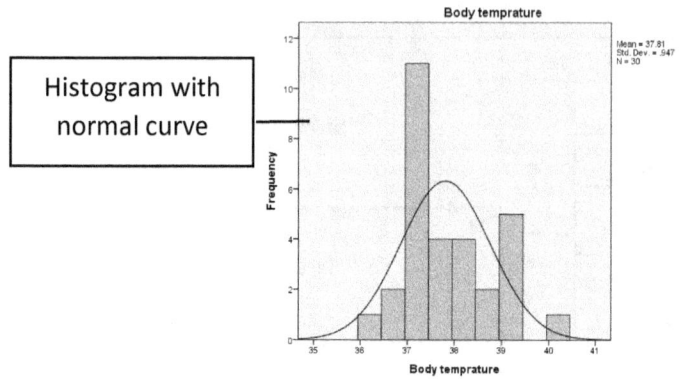

Pie chart

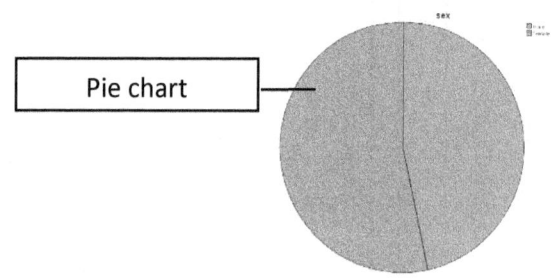

Frequency table

sex

		Frequency	Percent	Valid Percent	Cumulative Percent
Valid	male	14	46.7	46.7	46.7
	female	16	53.3	53.3	100.0
	Total	30	100.0	100.0	

Output of SPSS for Explore option

Descriptives

			Statistic	Std. Error
Body temprature	Mean		37.81	.173
	95% Confidence Interval for Mean	Lower Bound	37.45	
		Upper Bound	38.16	
	5% Trimmed Mean		37.77	
	Median		37.50	
	Variance		.897	
	Std. Deviation		.947	
	Minimum		36	
	Maximum		40	
	Range		4	
	Interquartile Range		2	
	Skewness		.637	.427
	Kurtosis		-.532	.833

Tests of Normality

	Kolmogorov-Smirnov[a]			Shapiro-Wilk		
	Statistic	df	Sig.	Statistic	df	Sig.
Body temprature	.172	30	.023	.921	30	.029

a. Lilliefors Significance Correction

Tests for normality: Kolmogorov-Smirnov for large samples (n over 30 at least) – Shapiro-Wilk for smaller samples

SPSS denotes "p value" as "Sig." as short for significance.

Significant test (p value below 0.05) means that the variables is NOT normally distributed.

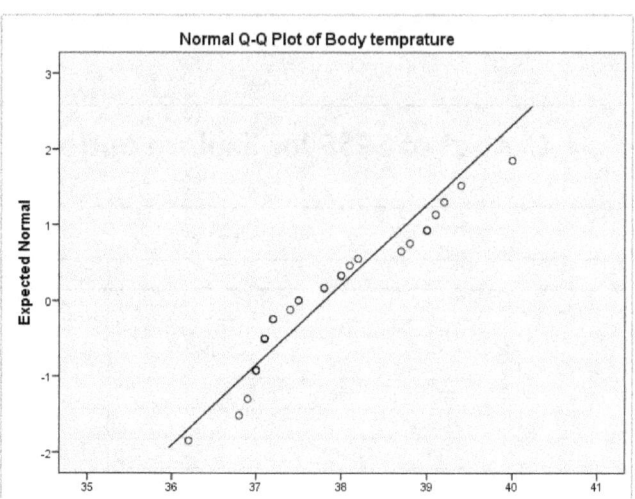

Q-Q plot asses the normal distribution of the variable, the line represent the ideal normal distribution. When the dots (cases) approach the line, it means the distribution approach normal, and vice versa.

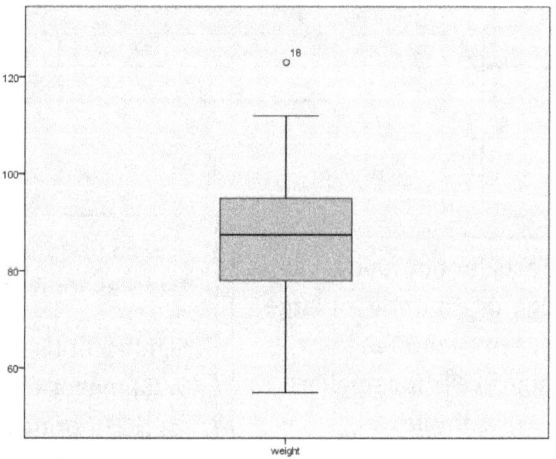

Box-whisker plot defines outliers as a dot either above or below the whisker. Also you can now initial information about normal distribution if the areas of the 4 quartiles are nearly equal.

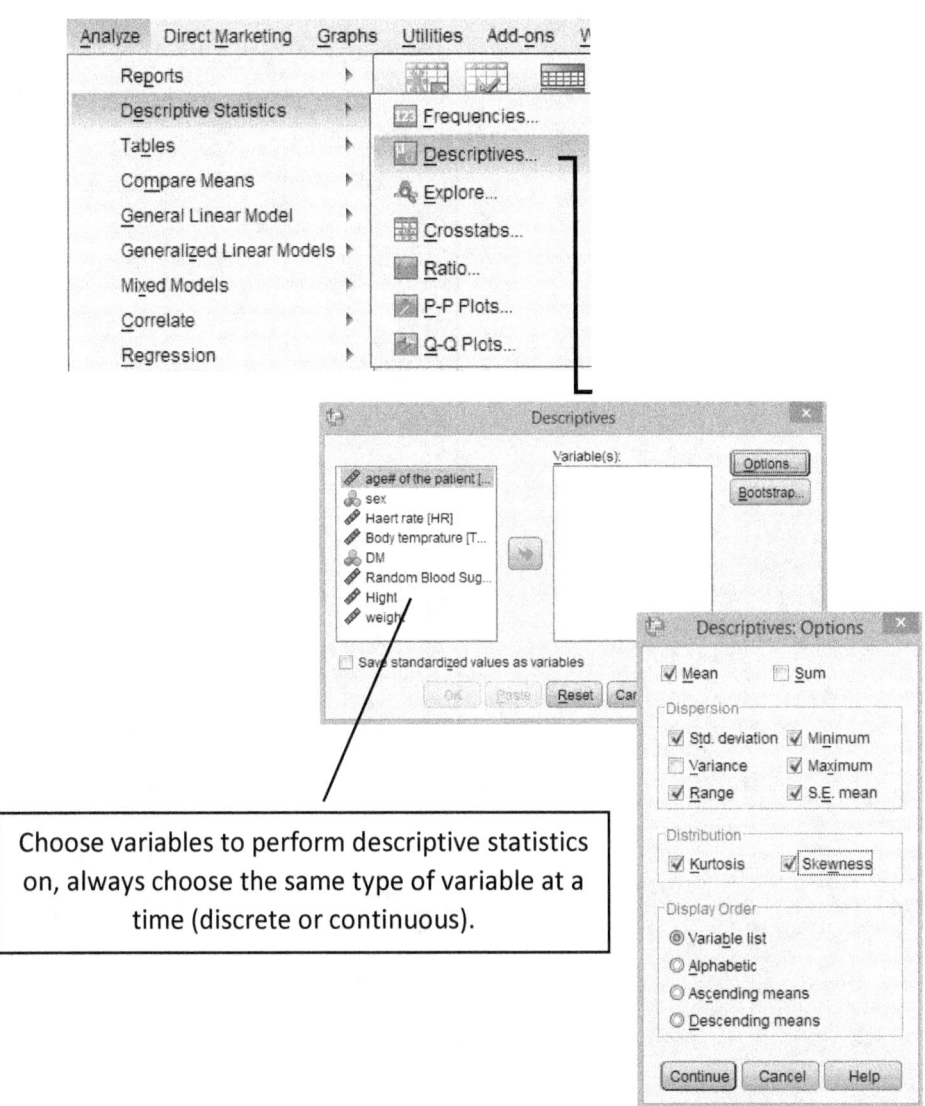

Choose variables to perform descriptive statistics on, always choose the same type of variable at a time (discrete or continuous).

Output of SPSS for Descriptives option

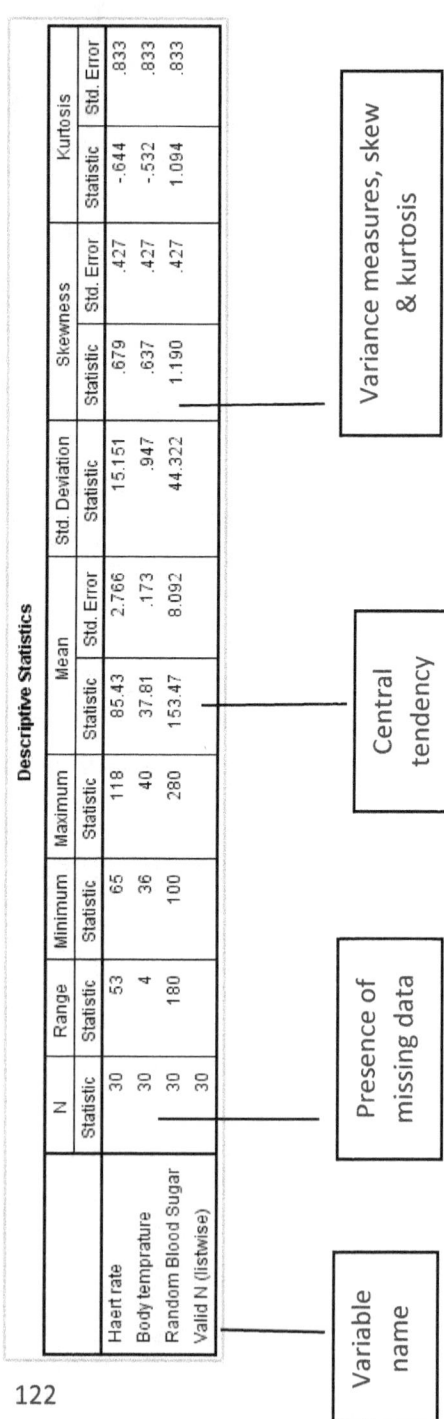

Descriptive Statistics

	N	Range	Minimum	Maximum	Mean		Std. Deviation	Skewness		Kurtosis	
	Statistic	Statistic	Statistic	Statistic	Statistic	Std. Error	Statistic	Statistic	Std. Error	Statistic	Std. Error
Haert rate	30	53	65	118	85.43	2.766	15.151	.679	.427	-.644	.833
Body temprature	30	4	36	40	37.81	.173	.947	.637	.427	-.532	.833
Random Blood Sugar	30	180	100	280	153.47	8.092	44.322	1.190	.427	1.094	.833
Valid N (listwise)	30										

Variable name

Presence of missing data

Central tendency

Variance measures, skew & kurtosis

122

Correlation

Perform Scatter plot, bivariate correlation

Analyze > Correlate > Bivariate

Insert variable

For ordinal vs. scale or 2 scale not normally distributed

For 2 scale normally distributed

Graphs > Legacy dialogs > Scatter/dots plot

2 variables

More than 2

Dependent

Independent

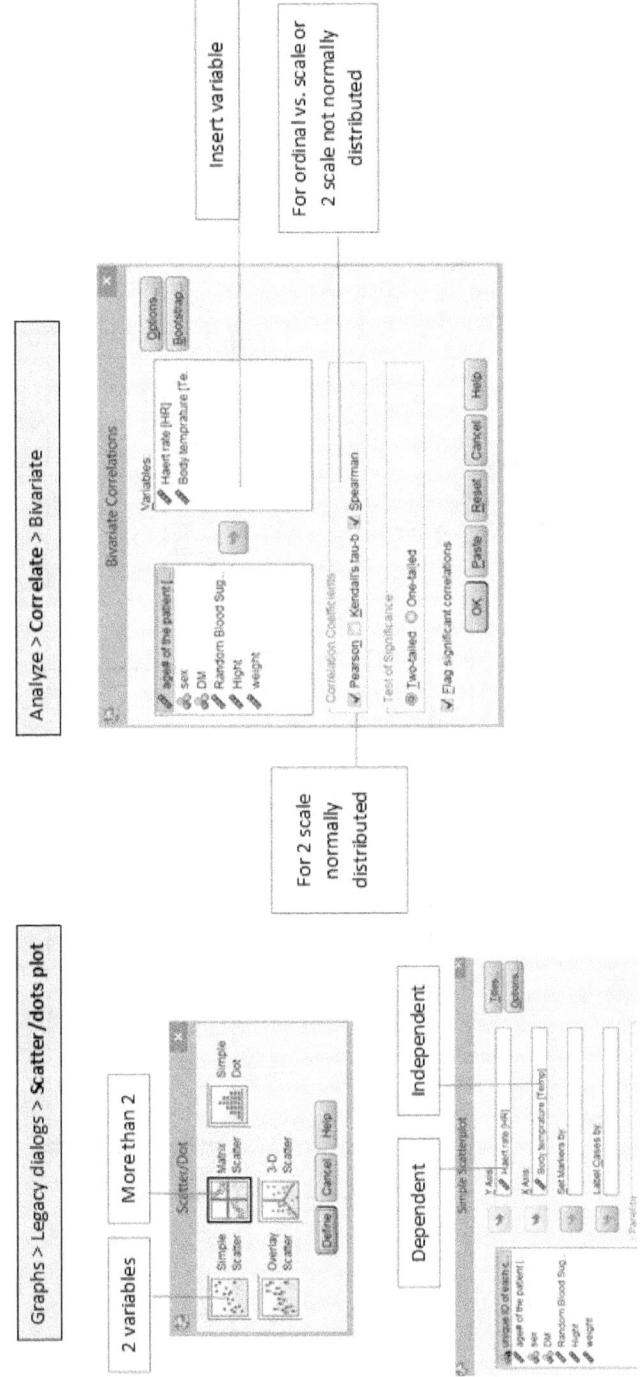

Output for correlation test

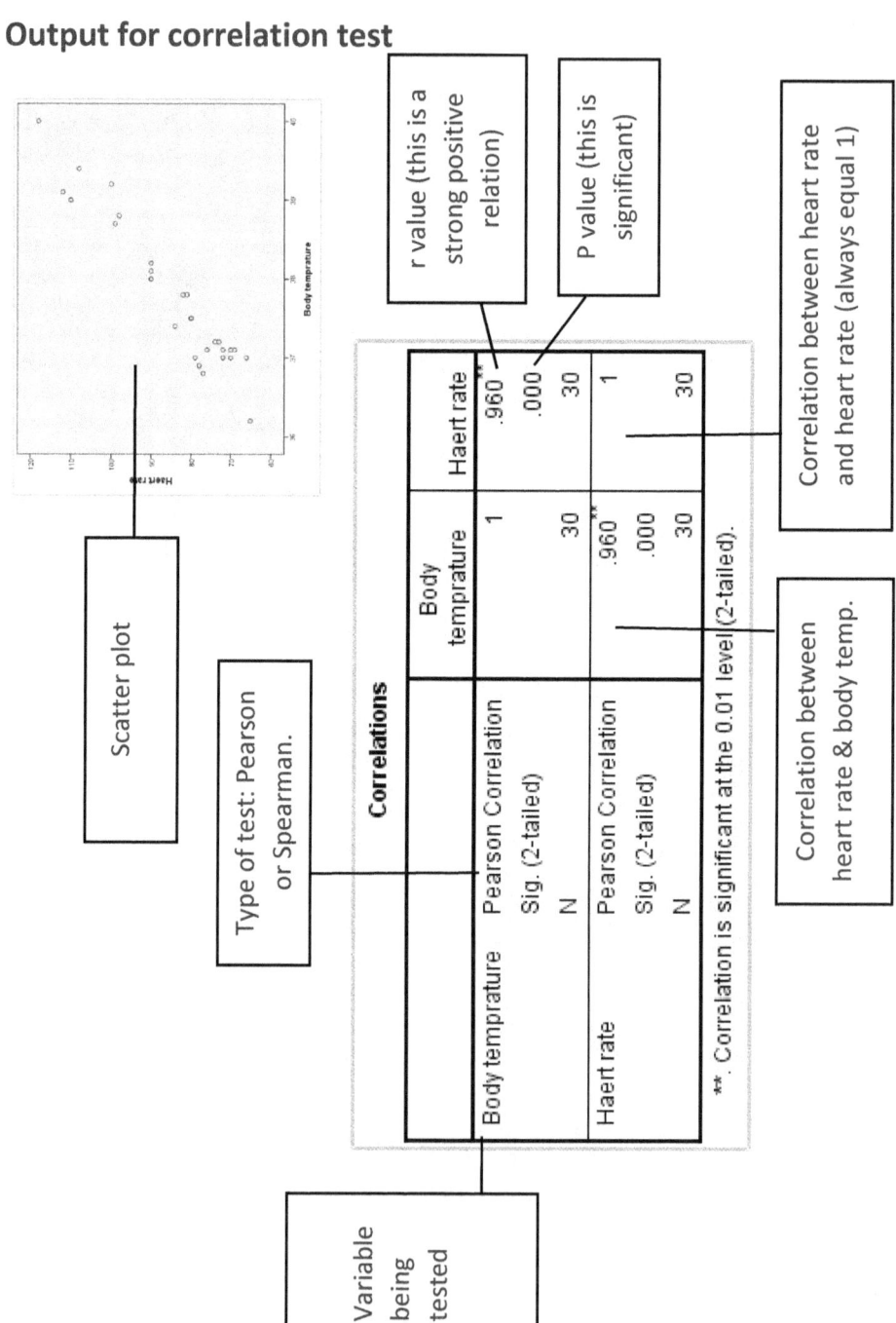

Part 2
Scientific Publications Handling

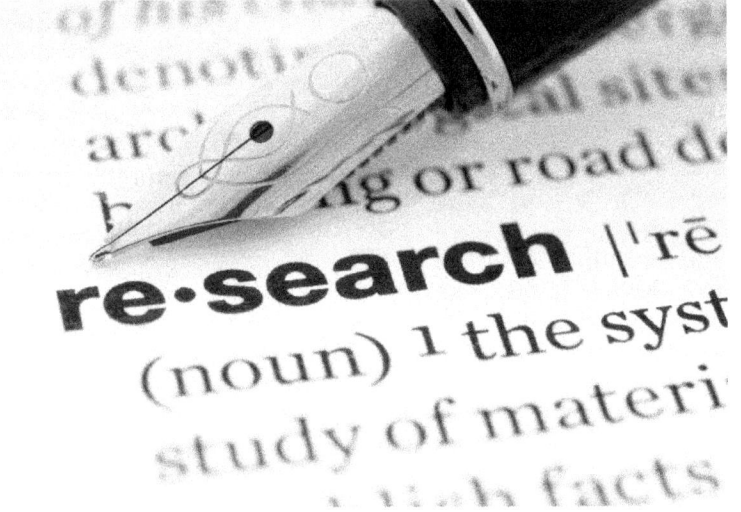

Explore the scientific writing process starting with a look on useful research techniques like literature review, then a detailed description of the original manuscript, key language hints and finally the publishing process landmarks.

Chapter 9: Literature Review: Sources of Medical Information

Learning objectives:

- Personal Contact, Books, Journals, Websites and Grey literature
- Bibliographic databases
- Search engines and its interfaces Features

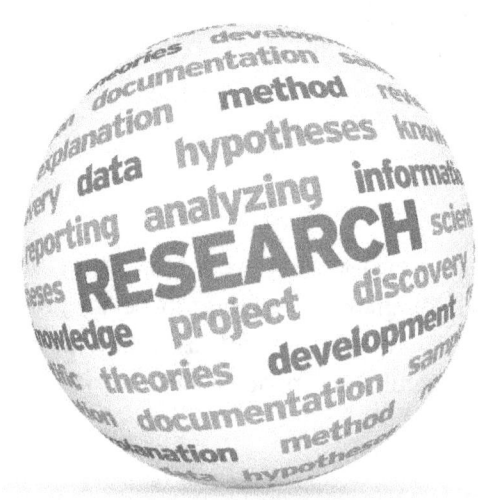

According to studies on information seeking behavior, textbooks and personal contact followed by journal articles are the most widely used sourced of clinical information.

Personal Contact is not limited to asking senior staff in the hospital or institute you are working in. It can also be achieved through emails, letters, telephone calls and conferences.

Books are available as hard copies through libraries or soft copies through online websites and libraries. Examples of such online libraries include MD consult Books, Oxford Medical Handbooks. Most of these websites require subscription.

Medical Journals are the third most commonly used source of medical information. Every medical journal has its own website and tries to link itself to multiple bibliographic database and search engines. Subscription can be done to the journal or to the whole publishing company. This allows receiving issue alert and newsletter of updates of the publication. Access to full-text-article is not allowed except for open-access journals or articles. Otherwise you will have to purchase the article to get the full text. A physician must be aware of the influential journals in his field and tries to keep pace with the updates of the issues of these journals.

Bibliographic databases

This is an indexed list of published information. This list is updated using special software and presented in many forms "printed, online and on CDs". Bibliographic databases can be searched using search engines or interfaces. Most medical journal and literature seek popularity and wide-spread access to readers via being linked to multiple and famous databases. The most famous and well-known databases are: Medline Database, Cochrane Database and Embase. Database may contain raw articles without previous evaluation from medical experts or it can be limited to pre-appraised articles.

Medline database is a bibliographic database that is compiled by the National Centre for Biotechnology Information (NCBI) of the U.S. National Library of Medicine (NLM). It contains over 14 million records from about 4,800 publications (mainly medical journals) from the 1950s to today. New citations are added daily.

Cochrane library contains many databases. The Cochrane Database of Systematic Reviews (CDSR) contains database for already-finished systematic reviews and also for the protocols of the systematic reviews under research. The Database of Abstracts and Reviews of Effectiveness (DARE) contains database of structured abstracts of high quality systematic reviews published in medical literature and also contains reference to reviews which will be helpful in building an effective background. The Cochrane Central Register of Controlled Trials [CENTRAL] is a database for articles reporting clinical trials. There are other databases in the

Cochrane library but the previous three are the most important ones.

Embase from Elsevier Life Science Solutions is an international biomedical database for biomedical researchers. It enables you to track and retrieve precise information on drugs and diseases from pre-clinical studies to searches on critical toxicological information.

AIDSLINE database: References the literature on AIDS back to 1980.

AMED database: Covers a range of complementary and alternative medicine including homeopathy, chiropractic, and acupuncture etc...

Search engines and interfaces Features in search engines

In order to search effectively, a researcher needs to be familiar with the database he uses by reading its guide, help pages (or tutorial) and checking examples available.

Although, they may differ in searching capacities and features, most databases have a basic search function and an advanced search function. Some databases have an intermediate search function.

Basic Search function:

The basic search box only searches one field. It is useful in determining the volume of the literature dealing with the topic or when searching an exact title.

Advanced Search function:

It allows more control to the user. Multiple search terms in multiple fields can be searched for simultaneously. It is used to know the large collection of the literature or when searching for a certain item as an author name or so.

Limits:

Many databases allow limiting the database by adding specified parameters as limiting the search by date, format, material type, language, or location.

Controlled Vocabulary "standardized vocabulary" "descriptors" "Subject headings":

Many databases use controlled vocabulary. It is similar to International Classification of Diseases (ICD9/10) codes. These are "preferred" words selected by specialists in information science and/or academic disciplines. Each word stands for a group of related words and concepts. Common controlled vocabularies in use are Library of Congress Subject Headings (LCSH) or Medical Subject Headings (MeSH), but any database can create its own controlled vocabulary. Obviously, controlled vocabulary requires periodical updating to keep up with the progress of science.

Advantages of searching via controlled vocabulary is it helps in searching related terms as they include synonyms, avoiding the problem of homonyms, searching unfamiliar terms and eliminating the spelling errors.

The Library of Congress Subject Headings (LSCH) list is listing over 280,000 subject headings. It is the most comprehensive list of subject headings and is the only one accepted as the worldwide standard.

Medical Subject Headings (MeSH) is created by the National Library of Medicine and used for PubMed (MEDLINE) article records. Over 24,000 descriptors are arranged in a hierarchical manner called the MeSH Tree Structures.

Thesaurus: A thesaurus is "an alphabetically arranged lexicon of terms comprising the specialized vocabulary of an academic discipline or field of study, showing the logical and semantic relations among terms, particularly a list of subject headings or descriptors used as preferred terms in indexing the literature of the field" (Reitz, 2004-6).

Keywords "Free-text searching":

These are words that may be found in the title, subject headings (descriptors), contents note, abstract, or text in a bibliographic database. Phrase searching can be done by putting words between quotation marks. Using quotation marks in PubMed prevents the MeSH matching. Searching via keywords is easy, less time-consuming and can keep up with new terms and innovations.

Proximity search is a feature supplied by some search engines. Proximity query operators include "NEAR, FOLLOWED BY, SENTENCE, Adj., etc.." Some search engines allows defining the number of words between the words. Proximity search is more important when the number of keywords is more than two.

Other Features:

These features may distinguish a database from another. Examples of these features are searching within results, analyzing results, search history, search by taxonomic data and showing related articles and links.

Truncation and wildcards:

Truncation symbols "wildcards" are used to search variant forms of a word as a single search concept rather than using variable keywords as individual concepts. This is done by replacing some characters in the beginning, middle or end of a word by a truncation symbol.

Truncating too early at the end of the word can broaden the search to unrelated topics. Common truncation symbols included the *, #,$, and ?.

Combining terms (Boolean searching):

This allows a searcher to connect words using the Boolean operators "AND" "OR" and "NOT" to broaden or narrow the search concept. The Boolean operator 'OR' is used to expand the search to include all records that contain either term. Truncation is not possible in these circumstances.

The Boolean operator 'AND' is used to narrow the search results by confining results to records containing both search terms. The Boolean operator 'NOT' is used to eliminate records related to unwanted concept in the search process.

Websites:

Some websites are assigned to a medical association or organization. These websites contain reports of value for physicians and clinicians in the field.

Examples: WHO, American Diabetes Association, Canadian Diabetes Association.

Grey literature:

Grey literature is a term used in library and information science. It refers to informally published written material. They are usually not found via conventional search channels. This includes dissertations, theses, patents, reports from governmental agents, working papers of research groups and conference proceedings.

For example: The URL (http://www.eulc.edu.eg/) takes you to the dissertations and theses from the Egyptian universities.

Search engines URL addresses	
Search Engine	URL
PubMed	http://www.ncbi.nlm.nih.gov/pubmed
Google Scholar	http://scholar.google.com
Library of Congress	http://www.loc.gov/index.html
Cochrane Library	http://www.thecochranelibrary.com/view/0/index.html
OVID	http://www.ovid.com
ScienceDirect	http://www.sciencedirect.com/
Scopus	http://www.scopus.com/
Uptodate	http://www.uptodate.com/home
Dynamed	https://dynamed.ebscohost.com/

Search engines information and details

Search engine Interface	Databases	Provided by	Articles	Text	Subscription
PubMed	Medline and Premedline	National Library of Medicine	Raw	Available or not	Not needed
Google Scholar	Web-based search engine	Google Inc.	Raw	Available or not	Not needed
Library of Congress	Database of books	Library of Congress	Raw		Not needed
Cochrane Library	Cochrane databases	The Cochrane Collaboration	Pre-appraised	Available	Not needed
OVID	AIDSLine, BioethicsLine, Medline, Premedline, CINAHL etc.	OVID	Raw		Needed
Science Direct		Elsevier publication	Raw	Available	Needed
Scopus		Elsevier publication	Raw	Available	Needed
Up-to-date		Wolters Kluwer Health	Pre-appraised	Available	Needed
Dynamed			Pre-appraised	Available	Needed

Chapter 10: Literature Review: Medical Search

Learning objectives:

- How to conduct a search in the literature?
- General Search Strategies
- Critical appraisal of search results

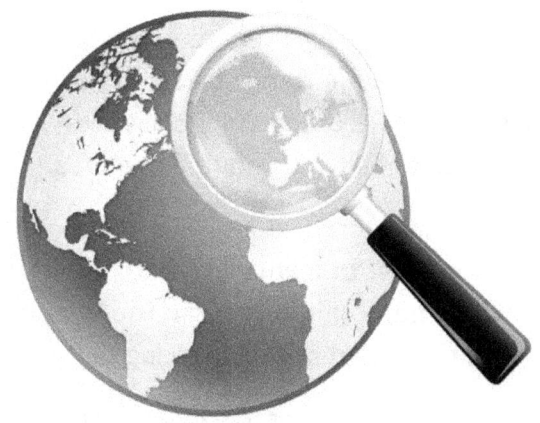

How to conduct a search in the literature?!

As stated before, textbooks and personal contact followed by journal articles are the most widely used sources of clinical information. Although the use of internet as a source of information has dramatically increased, the efficiency of searching has not grown apace.

There are many barriers that stand in the way of health professionals during their search for information in their field. The most important obstacles are: lack of time, lack of facilities, and lack of searching skills, lack of motivation and -perhaps worst of all- information overload.

The medical literature is like a jungle. In fact, the hardest task now is to actually locate the information required from the flood of information. The first question you must answer is that: what are you looking for?!

A searcher may approach medical (and, more broadly, health science) literature for three broad purposes: browsing to keep current and to satisfy our intrinsic curiosity; looking for answers, perhaps related to questions that have occurred in clinic or that arise from individual patients and their questions; surveying the existing literature, perhaps before embarking on a research project.

Browsing to keep current and to satisfy our intrinsic curiosity can be achieved by using alerting services to let us know when a new issue has been published and even tell us if articles matching our interest profile are in that issue. We can have RSS feeds of articles from particular journals or on particular topics sent to our email addresses or our iPhone or personal blogs, and we can participate in Twitter related to newly published papers. Almost every journal has links from its home page allowing at least one of these social networking services. These technologies are changing continuously.

Searching for an answer is to some extent an easy job. When we find that trustworthy information, it is OK to stop looking – we don't need to beat the bush for absolutely every study that may have addressed this topic.

Surveying: The purpose here is less to influence patient care directly than to identify the existing body of research that has addressed a problem, clarify the gaps in knowledge and explain your research findings. Multiple relevant databases need to be searched systematically, and citation chaining needs to be employed to assure that no stone has been left unturned.

General Search Strategies

Step 1: Create a research question

You can use a broad research question to get idea about the quantity of literature on the topic or to get new search ideas and key words or when you think that your question was not exclusively studies alone. The narrower the research questions, the more limited the search results become.

Step 2: Choose your resources:

- Manual search in the library of your institute.
- Searching public, private or specialized bibliographic databases.
- Grey literature.
- Asking an expert.
- Searching resources of macromedia.
- Search web reports.

Step 3: Break your question into concepts.

- Question of intervention? PICO system[9]
- Question of etiology and risk factors?
- Question of frequency and prevalence?

9
P   Population/patient
I   Intervention/indicator
C   Comparator/control
O   Outcome

- Question of diagnosis, prognosis and prediction?

Step 4: Put keywords and controlled vocabulary to every concept.

Step 5: Choose bibliographic databases and search engines appropriate to your topic.

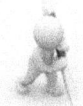 *Recent researches concluded that the use of a single search tool can lead to loss of up to 70 % of the relevant citations in some cases. Hence, using many search tools is recommended (Bajpai et al, 2011).*

Step 6: Conduct the search

- Use Boolean searching (Combine search synonyms with "OR" and combine search concepts with "AND").
- Use phrases for searching certain idea.
- Make advantage of the search features in the database or search engine you are using.
- Change approaches as necessary
- Continue to identify applicable keywords and controlled vocabulary to go back and check in the selected database(s) and other resources.
- Checking more than one can be very useful to pick up unique titles.
- Check references of the articles you find for detection of relevant articles.

- Identify key journals and perform a manual search on their issues.
- Collect your search results after removing duplicates. Using a citation manager (e.g. RefWorks and EndNote) may help.

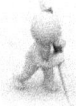

Remember that: The process of literature search and review should be systematic, explicit and reproducible.

Critical appraisal of search results

Critical appraisal is the process of carefully and systematically examining research to judge its trustworthiness, and its value and relevance in a particular context (Burls. 2009). Critical appraisal is an important step during literature review to overcome information overload and to get rid of irrelevant clinical studies.

It is a great frustration to find some persons who are supposed to be part of the scientific community who take their information from news articles and internet forums, or those who are not familiar with changes in the scientific paradigms, or those who don't know the levels of evidence or those who can't determine the scope of experimental method.

One of the major pre-requisites for evaluating a paper is being familiar with types of study designs and levels of evidence in quantitative studies.

Study Design

Qualitative Studies

Deal with non-numerical data which cannot be expressed in numbers. This includes observational studies, in depth interviews, focus group and documentary study.

Quantitative Studies

Deal with numerical data that can be converted into numbers.

- **Case report** and **case series report**: Report a single or a series of patients respectively. These are no control groups.
- **Case control study:** starts from the outcome to explore effect of exposure and possible links through the study of two groups; one with the outcome and the other without the outcome. It is very useful in causation research.
- **Cross-sectional survey:** Observation of a defined population at a single point in time or time interval. Exposure and outcome are determined simultaneously. It is very useful in diagnosis and screening research.
- **Cohort study:** Starts from the exposure to explore its effect on the outcome and possible links through the study of two groups; one received the exposure and the other without the exposure. It is very useful in causation research as well as prognosis research.
- **Randomized Controlled Trial (RCT):** A clinical trial in which participants are randomly allocated to a test treatment and a control. It is the gold standard in testing the efficacy of an intervention.
- **Systematic review:** Is a formalized and stringent process of combining the information from all relevant studies of the same health condition; these studies are usually clinical trials of the same or similar treatments but may be observational studies. It has the advantages of refinement and reduction, efficiency, generalizability, reliability and power. This is different from review article (which is a summary of

more than one paper on a specific topic, and which may or may not be comprehensive).

- **Meta-analysis:** A particular type of systematic review that focuses on the numerical results. The main aim of a meta-analysis is to combine the results from individual studies to produce, if appropriate, an estimate of the overall or average effect of interest.
- **Point of care resources:** These are like electronic textbooks or detailed clinical handbooks, but explicitly evidence-based and continuously updated.
- **Practice guidelines:** Are systematically arranged statements to outline appropriate health care for specific clinical circumstances. The panel developing the guideline includes representatives from all relevant disciplines, including patients, and the recommendations are explicitly linked to the evidence from which they are derived. One should bear in mind who put the guidelines and for what purpose. If the initial purpose of the guideline was very different from the purpose you want to use it for, it may not match your needs.

Useful websites for systematic reviews	The Cochrane Library www.cochrane.org
	The Campbell Collaboration www.campbellcollaboration.org
	The Centre for Evidence-Based Medicine www.cebm.net
	The NHS Centre for Reviews and Dissemination www.york.ac.uk/inst/crd
	Bandolier www.medicine.ox.ac.uk/bandolier
	PubMed Clinical Queries:
Sources of guideline in general	TRIP (Turning Research into Practice, http://www.tripdatabase.com)
	National Guideline Clearinghouse (NGC, http://www.guideline.gov/)
	National Institute for Health and Clinical Excellence (NICE, http://www.nice.org.uk/)
Sources for guidelines in a certain topics	Guidelines by the American Association for The Study of Liver Disease (AASLD): http://www.aasld.org/practiceguidelines/Lists/PG%20Content%20Query%20List/AllItems.aspx
	Guidelines by the European Association for the Study of the Liver (EASL): http://www.easl.eu/_clinical-practice-guideline
	Guidelines by the Canadian foundation of liver:http://www.liver.ca/liver-education-liver-research/resources-health-professionals/Clinical_Practice_Guidelines.aspx

Critical appraisal of Journal articles

Publication bias: Reviewers may be biased against unconventional techniques. Also, negative results don't (often) get published.

Authorship: Consider the institute to which the authors belong, issues of sponsorship and presence of conflict of interest.

Abstract quality: Don't depend on the abstract alone. Inaccuracies in the abstract can take multiple form including inconsistence between data in the abstract and in the manuscript, data in the abstract can't be found in the manuscript or the conclusion provided in the abstract is not covered in the manuscript.

Journal ranking and impact factors: Impact factor: a measure of the frequency with which the "average article" in a journal has been cited in a particular year or period. The impact factor is used to rank journals. In a given year, the impact factor of a journal is the average number of citations received per paper published in that journal during the two preceding years.

Methodological assessment: Prepared checklists are already available for critical appraisal of the content of an article.

Famous checklists	CASP www.sph.nhs.uk/what-we-do/public-health-workforce/resources
	SIGN Guideline Developers Handbook http://www.sign.ac.uk/guidelines/fulltext/50/annexc.html
	CEBMH http://cebmh.warne.ox.ac.uk/cebmh/education_critical_appraisal.htm

Critical appraisal of websites

- Consider the government, association, organization or other possible parties who would establish a medical website.
- Consider the intended audience and the purpose of site.
- Consider the sources of information.
- Consider if the data are up to date.

Chapter 11: Structure of the Original Manuscript

Learning objectives:

- What is the original manuscript?
- Sections of the original manuscript
- Aim of each section
- Tips on how-to-write each section

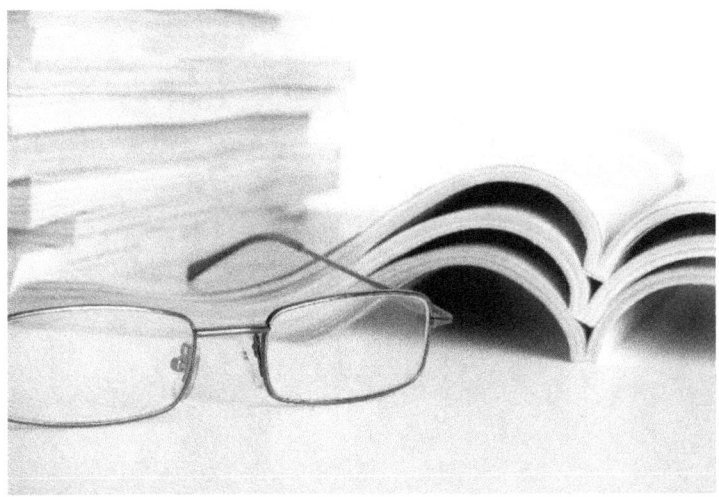

The original manuscript is the basic form of any scientific paper. Although the structure could vary according to the type of the paper that you are writing, the mainframe is usually constant. In this chapter we will go through each part of the original manuscript to describe its structure and to give hints on how to write it.

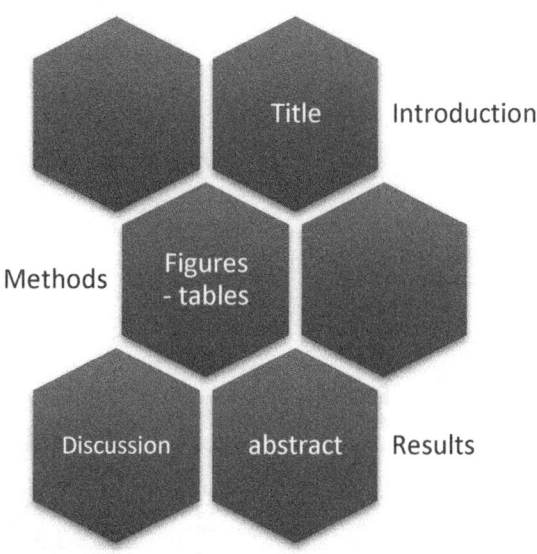

Tables and figures

Should be self-contained i.e. could be fully understood without any reference to the text of the manuscript. This because editors evaluate it first, also readers appreciate it first or even only.

Use the fewest number of tables and figure, don't repeat data in both tables and figures. And make sure that you have a sound justification for inserting each one of them.

When to use:

Figure: highlight important facts or results, visual impact, tell quick story, show trends and patterns.

Table: precise values, a lot of variables.

TABLES

Title: brief, with all information in the same keywords as the text.

Models the tables could be obtained from established tables in published paper or the guide to the author of each specific journal. *(but the most common pattern id to remove all gridlines except 3 horizontal ones: under title, under header and under data)*

Round all decimals to 0 or 1 according to the type of data. Put units of the measured variables.

Omit unnecessary columns (if p is significant in one or two variables put it in a footnote)

Footnotes: for acronyms and explanations statistical facts (P values, tests used), use the journal specific numbering format.

Figures

1. Primary evidence (x ray, pathology specimen)

2. Graph

3. Diagrams and drawing

Figure legend: brief title, explanation, panels, bars definitions, stat. Facts.

Results

Although the results section is not your ultimate victory in getting published and further recognized, it is an important part of your track. As it provides the outcome of your work. But remember to stick to the outcome and not its interpretation. So keep it to what you found only, not what you did (methods) or what you think this outcomes mean (discussions).

Deliver a summary of your data with citation of tables for details and describe major trends of these data in the text. Avoid repeating data described in tables and figures. But still you can repeat only highly significant numbers, or complement data in tables with percentages, or precise values not available in the table or figure.

Negative results are as important as positive results. So don't ignore them while writing down your results section. Actually negative results add to our scientific knowledge as much as positive results. Knowing what does not work or does not correlate is a step closer to knowing what does work or correlate. The following table offers a list of websites with good frames and checklist for how to present results according to various type of studies.

Table.[10] Reporting guidelines for various types of studies.
Consolidated Standards of Reporting Trials (CONSORT: www.consort-statement.org/)
Enhancing the Quality and Transparency of Health Research (EQUATOR; www.equator-network.org/home/)
Metaanalyses of Observational Studies in Epidemiology (MOOSE; JAMA 2000;283:2008–12)
Minimum Information about a Microarray Experiment (MIAME; www.mged.org/Workgroups/MIAME/miame_2.0.html)
Minimum Information for Biological and Biomedical Investigations (MIBBI; mibbi.org/index.php/Main_Page)
Minimum Information for Publication of Quantitative Real-Time PCR Experiments (MIQE; Clin Chem 2009;55:611–22)
Preferred Reporting Items for Systematic Reviews and Metaanalyses (PRISMA; www.prisma-statement.org/)
Standards for the Reporting of Diagnostic Accuracy (STARD; www.stard-statement.org/)
Strengthening the Reporting of Observational Studies in Epidemiology (STROBE; www.strobe-statement.org/)

---

[10] Annesley, T. M. (2010). Show your cards: the results section and the poker game. *Clinical chemistry*, *56*(7), 1066–70. doi:10.1373/clinchem.2010.148148

Options for presentation order of results.[11]

1. Chronological order: matching the methods section.

2. Grouping by topic or experiment: presenting each topic for all groups in a time *(e.g. survival among case and control groups then morbidity for each group. etc.)*

3. General to specific: demographic data for all groups, then specific data for each group alone. Most common pattern in clinical trial.

4. Most to least important.

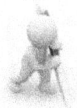 *A Grammar point: Use past tense as you are describing what you already found, but use present tense in (fig 2 shows, data suggests, we think...) because it still be present when he readers read it.*

---

[11] Previous reference

Methods

The aim of methods section is to provide enough information for anyone who wants to replicate the study. One of the most important fundamentals of scientific facts is being reproducible. That is why your research or experiment would be reproduced to confirm getting the exact same outcome. To ensure this will happen, your research must be carried out under the same conditions. So be clear and put down as much details about your methodology as you can.

Also methodology section enable reviewers and readers to evaluate the quality of your work. So give it its due attention to make sure that your research will be appreciated.

One more use of this section is for educational purposes. As a beginner scientist, you can learn a lot about research methodology from reviewing this section in various papers. You can use it while designing your research plan as a blue print.

Methodology section is the easiest part of your writing process. You are just reporting what you did throughout your research process. The table below can be used to as a guide to what information should be included. Mostly use passive voice as the subject – you – is always already known, also the passive voice brings the object (what was done) to the focus of attention in the beginning of the sentence. Use past tense as you are describing what was done in the past, except when you are referring to a table or a figure, you should use present tense. It is better to use diagrams or tables when they are saving a lot of words. One good examples for figures that do this is: the Participants flow diagram. (fig. below) If you tried to turn it into paragraph, it would be a long and rather boring one.

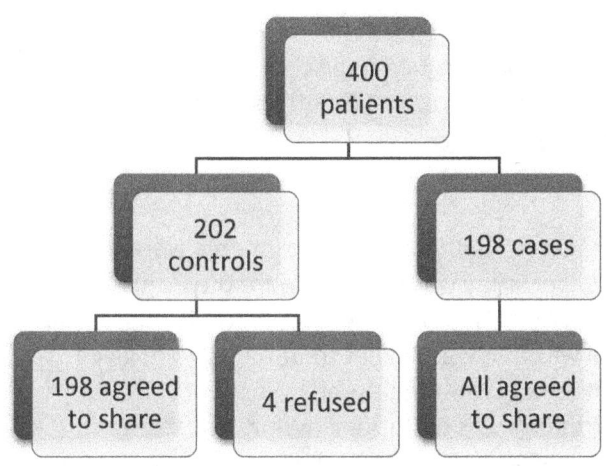

Table. [12]Who, what, when, where, how, and why questions to consider when writing the Methods section.
Who Who maintained the records? Who reviewed the data? Who collected the specimens? Who enrolled the study participants? Who supplied the reagents? Who made the primary diagnosis? Who did the statistical analyses? Who reviewed the protocol for ethics approval? Who provided the funding?
What What reagents, methods, and instruments were used? What type of study was it? What were the inclusion and exclusion criteria for enrolling study participants? What protocol was followed? What treatments were given? What endpoints were measured? What data transformation was performed? What statistical software package was used? What was the cutoff for statistical significance? What control studies were performed? What validation experiments were performed?
When When were specimens collected? When were the analyses performed? When was the study initiated?

---

[12] Annesley, T. M. (2010). Who, what, when, where, how, and why: the ingredients in the recipe for a successful Methods section. *Clinical chemistry*, *56*(6), 897–901. doi:10.1373/clinchem.2010.146589

When was the study terminated? When were the diagnoses made?
Where Where were the records kept? Where were the specimens analyzed? Where were the study participants enrolled? Where was the study performed?
How How were samples collected, processed, and stored? How many replicates were performed? How was the data reported? How were the study participants selected? How were patients recruited? How was the sample size determined? How were study participants assigned to groups? How was response measured? How were endpoints measured? How were control and disease groups defined?
Why Why was a species chosen (mice vs rats)? Why was a selected analytical method chosen? Why was a selected experiment performed? Why were experiments done in a certain order?

Introduction

Introduction is paving the road to your findings and outcome. It is the state of knowledge before your work, and the rational of carrying out your research. What is your research question or hypothesis, what knowledge gap that provoked it and what you did to fill this gap?

It is as it has a standard format, about 2 to 5 paragraphs (typically 3). It should follow the cone model converging from general to specific as follows.[13]

What is known where you state a quick background on the topic, then you move to what is unknown stating the limitation or knowledge gap in previous studies. After that state your hypothesis or research question in a clear statement like: We think that.... Or: We suggest that... Our aim was...etc. Now state your experimental or research approach, but not the exact methodology, just the outline. Finally show why it is unique and how it is going to fill the previously mentioned knowledge gap.

---

[13] Annesley, T. M. (2010). "It was a cold and rainy night": set the scene with a good introduction. *Clinical chemistry, 56*(5), 708–13. doi:10.1373/clinchem.2010.143628

Introduction section

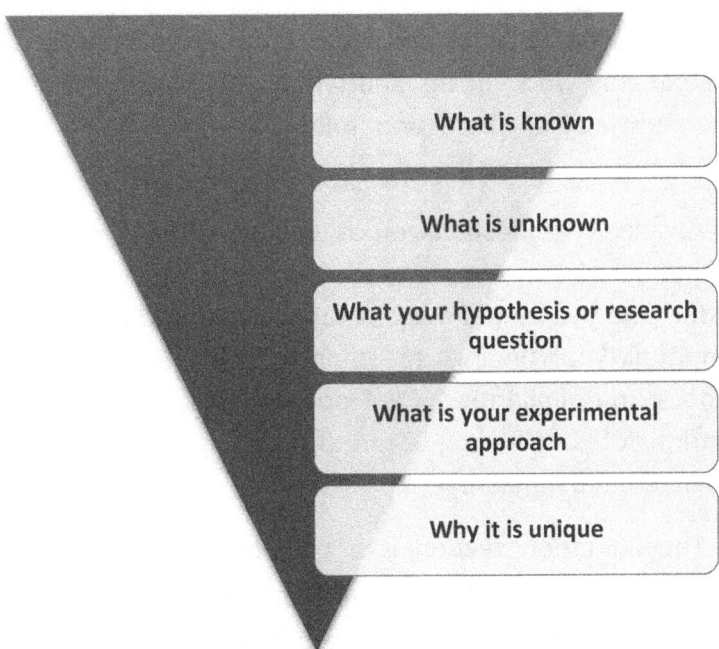

Discussion

This section is your argument that you did a good work, what this work means and what is its value to the general knowledge. Discussion follow an inverted cone model on contrary to the introduction, specific to general[14]

Answer the question you asked (hypothesis) = "we found that.....", then support your conclusion by evidence from your data by giving the big picture of your findings and by comparing your findings to others as well. Stating the differences and similarities. Give possible mechanisms or explanations of your findings. State if your findings support or challenge the paradigm.

The limitation section is a part of the discussion where you could defend your conclusion against anticipated criticism. Also you may recommend confirmatory or new studies to avoid your limitations or to expand the scope of your findings. The last sentence in your manuscript is the conclusion. Restate your main finding in clear concise words. This is the take home message of the article and probably the most important single sentence.

---

[14] Annesley, T. M. (2010). The discussion section: your closing argument. *Clinical chemistry*, 56(11), 1671–4. doi:10.1373/clinchem.2010.155358

Discussion Section

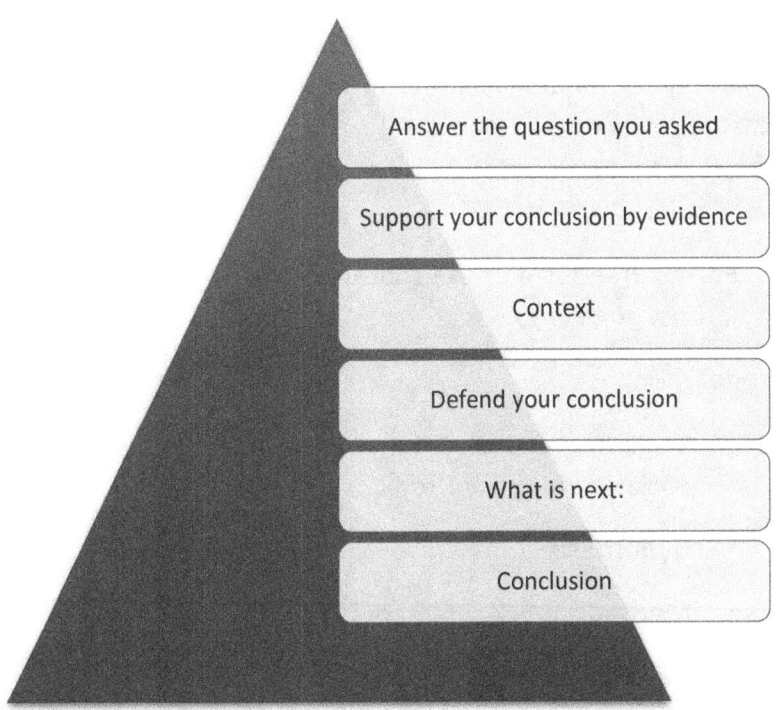

Abstract

Overview of the story with a highlight each section. It is concise but yet has to stand on its own *(as many readers will read only it)*. Its difficulty lays in its limited word count, as most journals restrict it to 150 to 200 words. So it take a lot of effort to summarize your entire article in such a short paragraph.

Forms: free form or the subtitles form. *According to the journal guidelines.*

Model

- **Background:** one sentence to explain the background of your topic

- **Hypothesis**

- **Methods:** quick summary

- **Results:** key only

- **Conclusion:** answer your question. And take home message

Table[15]. Characteristics of a well-written abstract.
Stands on its own without need to read the paper States the hypothesis, question, or objective of the study.
Completes the story by answering the hypothesis, question, or objective.

---

[15] Annesley, T. M. (2010). The abstract and the elevator talk: a tale of two summaries. *Clinical chemistry, 56*(4), 521–4. doi:10.1373/clinchem.2009.142026

Contains the same key words and terms as the title and the introduction.
Follows the correct style and format.
Follows the order of the main text (e.g., IMRAD)[16].
Stays within the allowed word count.
Does not contain information absent in the paper.
Does not make conclusions unsupported by the data.
Limits the use of abbreviations.
Does not include references.
Does not cite tables or figures

---

[16] The IMRAD format: Introduction, Methods, Results, and Discussion.

Citation

Choose the appropriate citation style according to the author guidelines of the journal you intend to publish in. APA (American Psychological Association) Style is one of the widely accepted styles for medical journals. The following is a summary of guidelines of how to cite according to APA style. Further information could be retrieved form Publication Manual of the American Psychological Association - American Psychological Association. Finally it much easier to use a software for retrieving and organizing your references.

In-text Citation with APA

The **author's last name** and **date of publication of the manuscript are included between parentheses,** and these items must match exactly the corresponding entry in the references list. eg (Robinson, 1998).

Major Citations for a Reference List/Bibliography[17]

Material Type	Reference List/Bibliography
A book in print	Baxter, C. (1997). *Race equality in health care and education.*Philadelphia: Ballière Tindall.
A book chapter, print version	Haybron, D. M. (2008). Philosophy and the science of subjective well-being. In M. Eid & R. J. Larsen (Eds.), *The science of subjective well-being* (pp. 17-43). New York, NY: Guilford Press.
An eBook	Millbower, L. (2003). Show biz training: Fun and effective business training techniques from the worlds of stage, screen, and song. New York: AMACOM. Retrieved from http://www.amacombooks.org/
An article in a print journal	Alibali, M. W. (1999). How children change their minds: Strategy change can be gradual or abrupt. *Developmental Psychology, 35,* 127-145.
An article in a journal without DOI	Carter, S., & Dunbar-Odom, D. (2009). The converging literacies center: An integrated model for writing programs.*Kairos: A Journal of Rhetoric, Technology, and Pedagogy, 14*(1).Retrieved from http://kairos.technorhetoric.net/
An article in a journal with DOI	Gaudio, J. L., & Snowdon, C. T. (2008). Spatial cues more salient than color cues in cotton-top tamarins (Saguinus oedipus) reversal learning. *Journal of*

[17] Citation Styles: APA, MLA, Chicago, Turabian, IEEE (2013, October 11). Retrieved December 10, 2013, from http://pitt.libguides.com/citationhelp

	Comparative Psychology, 122, 441-444. doi: 10.1037/0735-7036.122.4.441
Websites - professional or personal sites	*The World Famous Hot Dog Site.* (1999, July 7). Retrieved January 5, 2008, from http://www.xroads.com/~tcs/hotdog/hotdog.html
Websites - online government publications	U.S. Department of Justice. (2006, September 10). Trends in violent victimization by age, 1973-2005. Retrieved from http://www.ojp.usdoj.gov/bjs/glance/vage.htm
Emails (cited in-text only)	According to preservationist J. Mohlhenrich (personal communication, January 5, 2008).
Mailing Lists (listserv)	Stein, C. Chessie rescue - Annapolis, MD. Message posted to Chessie-L electronic mailing list, archived at http://chessie-l-owner@lists.best.com
Radio and TV episodes - from library databases	DeFord, F. (Writer). (2007, August 8). Beyond Vick: Animal cruelty for sport. In NPR (Producer), *Morning Edition.* Retrieved from Academic OneFile database.
Radio and TV episodes - from website	Sepic, M. (Writer). (2008, January 14). Federal prosecutors eye MySpace bullying case. In NPR (Producer), *All Things Considered.* Retrieved from http://www.npr.org/templates/story/
Film/Film Clips from website	Kaufman, J.-C. (Producer), Lacy, L. (Director), & Hawkey, P. (Writer). (1979). Mean Joe Greene [video file]. Retrieved from http://memory.loc.gov/mbrs/ccmp/meanjoe_01g.ram
Photograph (from book,	Close, C. (2002). *Ronald.* [photograph]. Museum of

magazine or webpage)	Modern Art, New York, NY. Retrieved from http://www.moma.org/collection/object.php?object_id=108890
Artwork - from library database	Clark, L. (c.a. 1960's). *Man with Baby.* [photograph]. George Eastman House, Rochester, NY. Retrieved from ARTstor
Artwork - from website	Close, C. (2002). *Ronald.* [photograph]. Museum of Modern Art, New York. Retrieved from http://www.moma.org/collection/browse_results.php?object_id=108890

Suggested order of writing

1. **Tables and figures**: this your data that tells your story.

2. **Results**: this is the summary of tables and figures.

3. **Methods:** can be written first but it is the most boring.

4. **Introduction:** unrelated to your story direct but you must know how it ends to be able to introduce it.

5. **Discussion:** the most sophisticated, leave it to the end.

6. **Abstract:** summary of all of the above, the last section to be written.

Chapter 12: Language

Learning objectives:

- Tips for scientific writing
- Common grammar pitfalls
- Summarizing
- Phases of writing

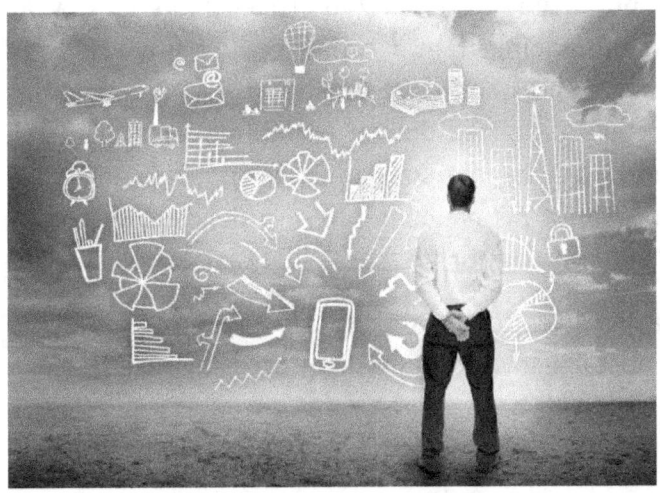

The language that you use represents the package that you wraps your ideas in. Although many think of language role as secondary in comparison to the data or scientific content of the paper, and others see it as just too boring or too complicated to learn, the truth is that many good papers was delayed or even rejected in the process of reviewing just because of its poor language.

When reviewers handle your paper they assume that you have dealt with the scientific details with maximal precision, but if they were stuck in broken sentences, weak words and misleading grammar, they could easily lose their way to your ideas, or at least doubts about your scientific methods could be raised due to a simple question: "If the author could not handle such a simple issue as language rules, what about his handling of more delicate issues like scientific methodology or statistical analysis?"

Paying attention to language rules is your gate to pass your first obstacle towards publishing. So make sure you pass it as safe and quick as possible.

We can divide language rules that you should master into the following categories:

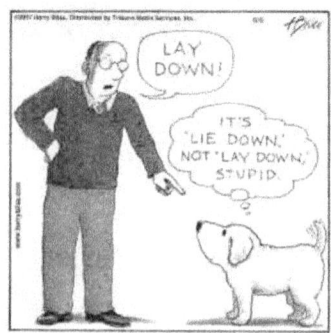

- Words and structures
- Grammar
- Punctuation
- Cutting the clutter

Words and structures

Spelling

Spelling mistakes are fatal, especially when frequent, this could reflects lack of attention to details or could be misleading if these mistakes change the meaning of the word. Use Autocorrect in Microsoft office to check your spelling, but be aware that the software usually do not afford correction for specialized medical terms. Those terms should be corrected manually.

Terminology

Using the most updated version of the scientific terms reflects that your knowledge is up-to-date and recent. Use the simplest possible – yet correct - alternative of the term.

Use online sources to verify medical terms such as: http://www.medicalterminologydb.com/

Or explore the Unified Medical Language System (UMLS) http://www.nlm.nih.gov/research/umls/quickstart.html created and maintained by the U.S. National medical library.

Capitals

The first word of a new sentence starts with a capital letter. Acronyms are written in capital letters too. And finally the names of persons and places start with a capital letter.

Distance between verb and subject (buried verb)

Keep a short distances between the subject (at the beginning of the sentence) and its verb. Do not insert a lot of description phrases in between. When necessary, split those sentences into shorter ones.

Do not use nouns for verbs

Verbs make your sentences more dynamic and less boring. Avoid the "ing" or "tion" overuse whenever possible.

Grammar

Tenses

Methods and results sections are usually written in the past tense. On the other hand, discussion and introduction sections are usually written in the present tense.

Singular or plural

Present tense "s" when the subject is singular.

Always check for match the following Verbs: *(be – have – do)*.

Active or passive

Always use the active voice throughout your manuscript as a general rule except in methods section use passive voice.

Affect/Effect

Diuretics affect ABP (verb)

Diuretics have an effect on ABP (noun)

Punctuation

These marks are the traffic lights of your text. They help the reader to better understand your ideas. Also they are used to vary sentences structure between short and long ones.

Colon :	• for definition, list, quote, and conclusion.
Semicolon ;	• joins 2 separate idea that should be linked. Also to separate items in the list with a higher power of separation (*e.g. internally, 5 items; externally, 3 items*)
Parenthesis ( )	• inserting a separate phrase inside the sentences that can be ignored.
Dash −	• dropping anything anywhere in the sentence, don't overuse it as it less formal.
Comma ,	• Items in list, phrases in one sentences.
Full stop .	• to end a full − Stand alone sentence.
Quotation " "	• Quotes of other authors.

Cutting the clutter

The clutter is simply the items that you can lose without affecting your process. Science is the continuous pursuing of exactness and accuracy. So always try to lose any aimless additives to your manuscript. Concise manuscripts are by far more attractive to both reviewers and readers, as neither of them have extra time for figures of speech and highly decorated phrases. Also you are usually bounded by a tight number of words defined by journal editors, and it is easy to overshoot this limit while writing. But here are some techniques to cut it back to the minimal word count.

Simply avoid the following:

• Dead weight words e.g. as it is well known, as we all know....etc.

• Long phrases that could be shortened

• Repetition

• Acronyms (unnecessary)

• Adverbs e.g. really, very, generally

• Negative phrases could be turned to shorter positive phrases of the opposite meaning: (instead of harmful; use: safe)

• There is, there are: Instead of: There are many factors that affect the environment, say: Many factors affect the environment.

Phases of the writing process

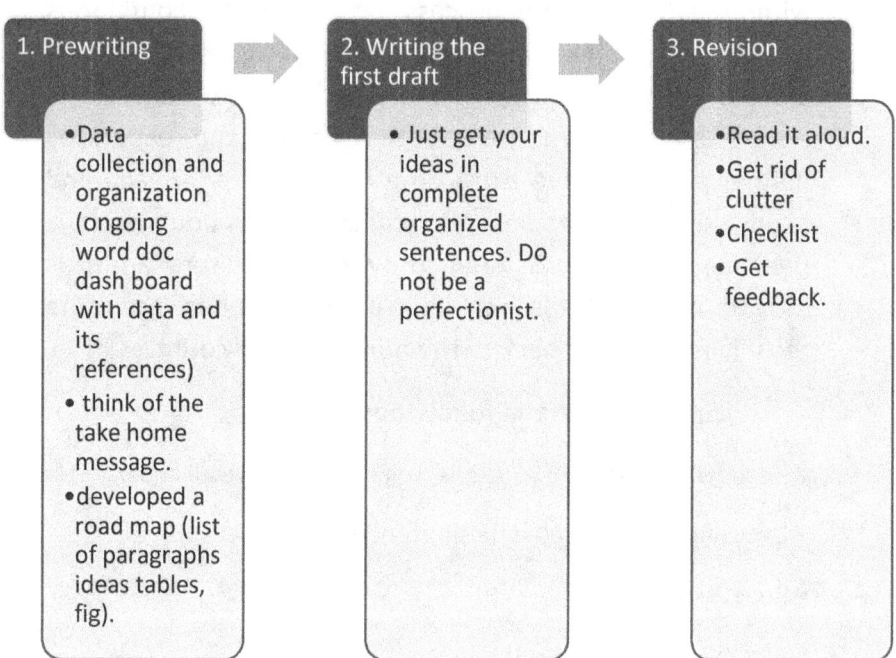

1. Prewriting

- Data collection and organization (ongoing word doc dash board with data and its references)
- think of the take home message.
- developed a road map (list of paragraphs ideas tables, fig).

2. Writing the first draft

- Just get your ideas in complete organized sentences. Do not be a perfectionist.

3. Revision

- Read it aloud.
- Get rid of clutter
- Checklist
- Get feedback.

Checklist

1. Check for consistency	No contradiction
	No false or inaccurate information
2. Verb check	buried verbs
	Passive voice
	Weak
	Verb to be
3. Numerical consistency	Number from abstract, text, figures all match.
4. References.	Make sure that the ref. indicated the fact you tell (no ref to nowhere) Revise ref. form and numbering.

Chapter 13: Getting Published

Learning objectives:

- Plagiarism
- Tips for choosing a journal to submit your manuscript to
- Manuscript editing
- Online submission process

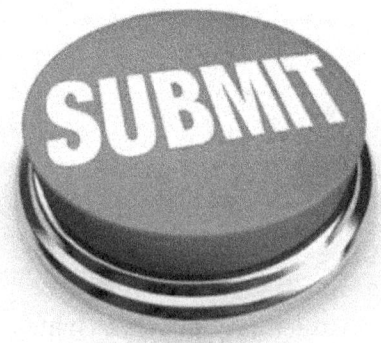

In this chapter we will explore the process of getting your manuscript published. While it may seem such a big and sophisticated task, it is really not that big. It is as simple as following some rules. Here is the rules.

Rule #1: avoid plagiarism, play it safe.

The definition of plagiarism is: "The act of using another person's words or ideas without giving credit to that person: the act of plagiarizing something."[18]

Simply, plagiarism is a crime. It is hardly go undetected as most journals use electronic plagiarism detectors that can compare your text to published works. Any significant match without proper citation will lead to dangerous consequences. First of all, your manuscript will be rejected, then you will be black-listed in this journal (and all related journals of the same publisher). Also you may be reported to your institution as a plagiarizer for further punishment. Bottom line: DO NOT PLAGIARIZE!

How to avoid plagiarism?

When using other authors works you should either quote or paraphrase.

Quoting:

It is using the same words of the authors after putting them between quotation marks (""). Then put the reference in the proper format.

---

[18] Plagiarism. 2014. In *Merriam-Webster.com*. Retrieved November 8, 2014, from http://www.merriam-webster.com/dictionary/plagiarism

Paraphrasing:

It means that you write the ideas or the results of the author but *in your own words* and without quotation marks. While quoting seems easier, you cannot put all the material that you use in your manuscript between quotation marks. If you do so, you will not be writing a manuscript, you will be just collecting other authors' words. Certainly rejected from publishing.

When paraphrasing, do not just change some words from the source manuscript to their synonyms. You must change the structure of the sentence itself. This is because if you just copy-pasted a text from a source (without quoting) and citing it, you will be giving the author credit for the science within the text, but stealing his writing style.

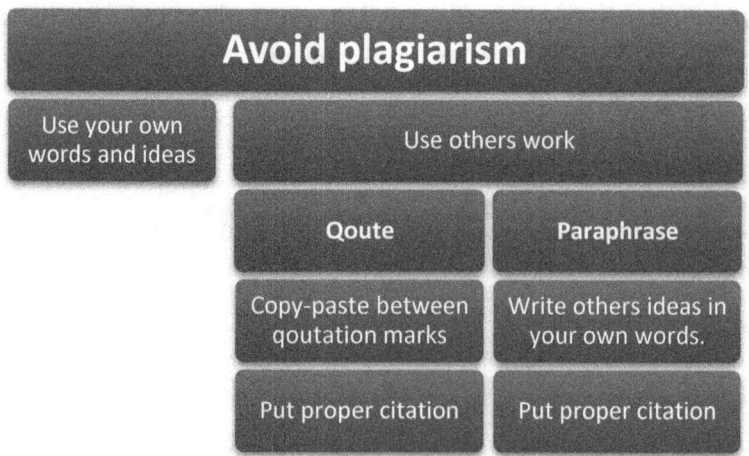

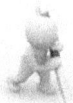

A lot of anti-plagiarism software and website are available on-line for free, Google it.

Rule #2: choose your journal

When coming to choosing the journal that you will submit your manuscript to, it is wise to follow the following tips to maximize your chances of getting published.

Title:

The journal's title must be relevant to your work. There are thousands of medical journals all over the world. All are reachable to your fingertips through the internet. Choose the most relevant title to your work. Also try the most specific.

For example if you have a manuscript about "outcome of surgery after left hemicolectomy for colorectal carcinoma". The following journals[19] are all suitable but in increasing chances:

1. World Journal of Surgery
2. World Journal of Gastrointestinal Surgery
3. International Journal of Colorectal Disease
4. Current Colorectal Cancer Reports

Content:

Explore the published articles in the journal you choose. Finding previous papers on related topics increases your chances of getting published as it shows the interest of the journal in this specific topic.

---

[19] These journals was found after search on www.springer.com

Types of accepted papers:

You can find this in the journal's website. Some journals do not accept certain types of papers, especially: case reports.

Reasonable impact factor:

Impact factor is an indicator of how effective this journal is in its field. It is calculated for each year by dividing the number of citations that the articles of journal got in the previous 2 years by the total number of papers published in the previous 2 years.

For example, 2014 impact factor is 2. This means that -on average- each article published in this journal in 2012 & 2013 was cited twice in the same period.

Choose a reasonable impact factor. Don't aim too high, yet don't underestimate your work by publishing it in a journal without even an impact factor.

Is there any fees??

Most peer-reviewed respected journal do not ask for fees. Yet there is the fees for the open access choice. This means that you can choose to pay a certain amount of money to make your article available for unregistered users of this journal. i.e. available for free to all internet users. The benefit you get is that your article can get more audience and in turn more citation and more impact. If you didn't choose this, you will still get published.

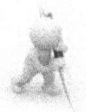 *It is good idea to submit your manuscript to the journals that appeared frequently in your references list. This may increase your chances, as it shows that the journal is interested in your topic. Also this may encourage the journal to publish your paper to increase its impact factor.*

Rule #3: play by the rules

Each journal has specific rules about submitting a manuscript. These rules can be found in a text titled: guide for authors, information for authors or any similar title. It is usually a short text that should be read carefully to be able to follow its rules, otherwise you would be rejected before even reviewing your content.

Examples of the rules that are commonly similar among journal:

1. Use simple font (Arial or Times New Roman) of size 10 or 12.
2. Use double spacing of the paragraph lines. From the function: line and paragraph spacing in your word processor. Adjust it to: 2.
3. Create tables by "table function" not by Excel spread sheets.
4. Do not use space to create the indent in the beginning of paragraphs. Use "tab" button instead.
5. Create a title page with the following information:
   - Article title
   - Authors' names and affiliation

- Short (running) title
- 3-5 Keywords relevant to your topic
- Full contact details of the corresponding author

6. Download a certain form for copyright transfer and sign it then resend it with your manuscript. You may sign using recent version of Adobe© PDF readers.

Examples of the rules that may differ from journal to another:

1. Text limit. For the abstract between 200 and 250 words. For the whole manuscript between 1500 to 3000 words.
2. Type of abstract: structured or not.
3. Type of citation.

Where to find the previous rules?[20]

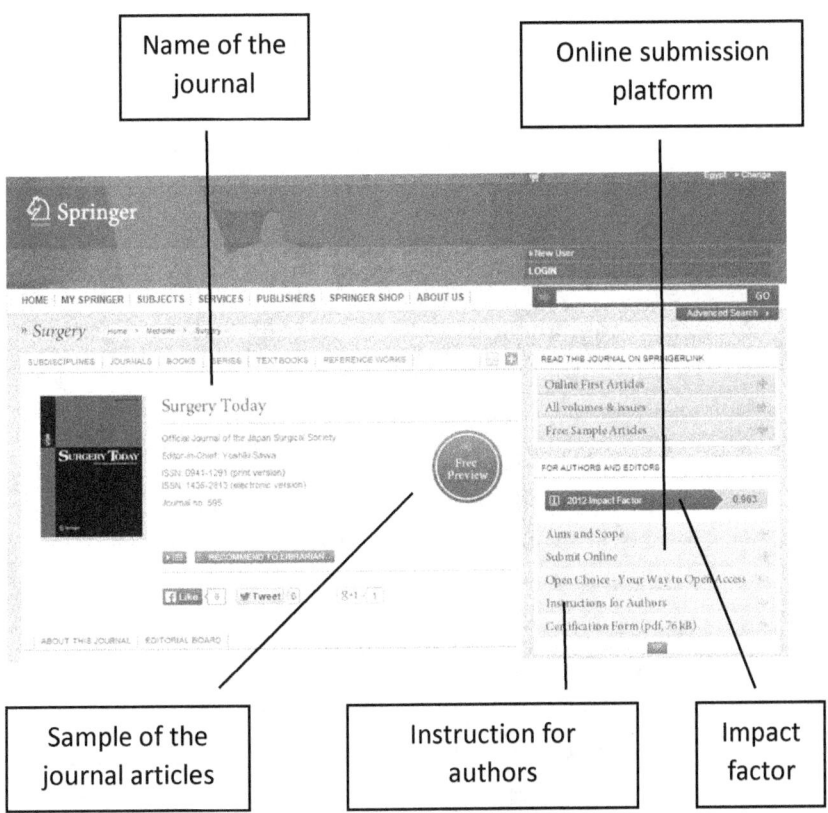

Name of the journal

Online submission platform

Sample of the journal articles

Instruction for authors

Impact factor

Rule #4: submit online

Almost all journals now use an electronic platform to receive manuscript for publishing. The mainframe of these platform is usually similar. Follow the instruction that appear with every step.

First of all create your account and set your password (for free). Then click on authors centers and follow the steps. The common steps are:

1- Log in
2- Enter the manuscript title, type and abstract
3- List the authors and co-authors
4- List the keywords
5- Add some specifications like a cover letter, reviewers' names and contacts – if requested.
6- Upload your files: usually the main document, the certificate form, tables and figures are uploaded separately.
7- Review the submission by downloading a pdf file in which all what you entered or uploaded are compiled. If no mistakes found, approve the submission. This is the only irreversible step.

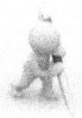

Keep a document with journals names you are registered in, along with your user names and passwords to keep track of your accounts.

Rule #5: keep track of your submission

Usually it takes weeks to get an answer from the journal about your submission. Try to resist your desire to login to the journal account twice daily to check. Be cool!!

You will get an email and the new status will appear in your journal account. The answer is either:

- **Accepted for publishing:** this is very rare. Don't wait for it.
- **Rejected without possible resubmission:** this means you are rejected by this journal. Check the reason. Is something wrong with your manuscript or just they are overwhelmed with manuscripts. Try another journal after fixing any issues.
- **Rejected with possible resubmission:** this is what you should wait for. It means you will probably get acceptance but after fixing some issues in your manuscript. The journal will send you a list of these issues. Read them carefully. Fix any issues if needed and send the manuscript again. Remember that you must enclose an email with the resubmission stating each issue and how you dealt with, either what changes you made or why you didn't change it (with a reasonable explanation of course).

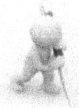
Do not get too depressed if you got multiple rejections. Established authors still may publish their articles in the fourth or fifth journal they contact. So cheer up! And keep trying!

Other books by the author

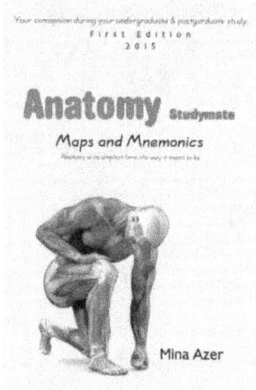

Anatomy Studymate: maps & mnemonics

Anatomy Studymate explains human anatomy the way it is meant to be explained, by maps and mnemonics instead of complicated pictures and long paragraphs.

This book has 5 chapters covering the main regions of the body: upper limb, lower limb, thorax, abdomen & pelvis and head & neck. It includes 235 topics further divided into 131 easy to remember mnemonics, 51 maps for a simple diagrammatic view of various anatomical structures, 30 tables summarizing almost all the muscles of the human body and finally 23 summary verses for extremely important topics that couldn't fit in one of the previous 3 categories, and yet cannot be ignored.

Available on amazon.com

http://goo.gl/B3LjSx **amazon**

ISBN-13: 978-1508887577

ISBN-10: 1508887578

www.ingramcontent.com/pod-product-compliance
Lightning Source LLC
Chambersburg PA
CBHW070855180526
45168CB00005B/1831